BEYOND SEPARATION

MEDICINE, ILLNESS AND SOCIETY

edited by W. M. Williams

Professor of Sociology and Anthropology
University College of Swansea

Hospitals, Children and their Families
The Report of a Pilot Study

Margaret Stacey (editor)
Rosemary Dearden   Roisin Pill
David Robinson

The Process of Becoming Ill

David Robinson

Going to See the Doctor

Gerry Stimson   Barbara Webb

Social Relations and Innovation
Changing the State of Play in Hospitals

David J. Hall

Beyond Separation

*Further Studies
of Children in Hospital*

Edited by

DAVID HALL

and

MARGARET STACEY

LONDON, BOSTON AND HENLEY

ROUTLEDGE & KEGAN PAUL

First published in 1979
by Routledge & Kegan Paul Ltd,
39 Store Street,
London WC1E 7DD,
Broadway House,
Newtown Road,
Henley-on-Thames,
Oxon RG9 1EN and
9 Park Street,
Boston, Mass. 02108, USA
Printed in Great Britain by
Redwood Burn Limited
Trowbridge & Esher

British Library Cataloguing in Publication Data

Beyond separation. – (Medicine, illness and society).
1. Children – Hospital care – Psychological aspects
I. Hall, David   II. Stacey, Margaret   III. Series
362.7'8'11   RJ242   79–40011
ISBN 0 7100 0163 0

Contents

Figures and Tables

Figures

Tables

Acknowledgments

There were seven researchers altogether working on the projects connected with children in hospital and we also employed various assistants in the way of observers, interviewers and secretaries. We were working in six different hospitals in three different regions. For all these reasons it is difficult to acknowledge fully our debt to the many willing people who helped us. These include the paediatric consultants, the orthopaedic consultants, other medical staff, the nurses, playleaders, the administrative, clerical and other staffs of the hospitals in which we studied. We have a special debt to the young patients who taught us so much and to their families who always co-operated willingly in our enquiries. We cannot acknowledge any of the authority staff, the hospital staff or the patients or their families by name because we wish to retain the anonymity of the hospitals and the staff and patients in them. This we promised. To all of them, nameless though they must be, our very grateful thanks for intrusions on their work, their home life and their suffering.

We would like to mention our debt to colleagues in the University College of Swansea: to those in the Psychology Department and especially Dr Mary Woodward for her guidance, and for her encouragement of the psychological studies; Professor W. M. Williams and colleagues in the Sociology Department, who were always supportive and helpful; colleagues in the Medical Sociology Research Centre and especially Professor R. Mapes who, by making Centre facilities available after the project was nominally finished, has helped us to complete our work, and Gail Eaton for help in reading drafts; the Department of Education for making facilities available for experimental work; the Computer Centre, particularly Mary Viner.

We would also like to thank Professor Peter Gray, Dr J. Bowlby and Professor H. R. Schaffer for help and comments on various drafts; the members of seminars and conferences – medical, nursing, psychological and sociological – for their comments on various papers we read to them; Mrs Bianca Gordon and members of her Children in Hospital Study Groups (run in association with the Hampstead Child Therapy Clinic, London, supported by the Grant Foundation, New York); the teachers who completed the Bristol Social Adjustment Guide; members of the Welsh Hospital Board and its staff, and especially those connected with the Working Party on Children in Hospital in Wales.

We would like to thank the interviewers and observers who helped us, often at unsocial hours, and all the secretaries who helped, including the secretarial staff of the Charles Burns Clinic and Tennal School, Birmingham, Lesley and Joan in the Sociology Department of the University of Warwick. Very special thanks to Vicky and June, the secretaries at the Centre, who stoically bore the brunt of the work.

Finally, we must thank the Department of Health and Social Security for funding the project and for their flexibility in its administration.

The responsibility for what we have finally written must rest on each of us who have contributed to the book.

The contributors and publishers would like to thank the following for permission to reproduce copyright material: National Foundation for Educational Research, for permission to reproduce Figure 2.1A, from E. Bene and J. Anthony, *Manual for the Family Relations Test*, London, 1957; the editors of the *Nursing Times* for permission to use material in ch. 5, published in *Nursing Times*, 14 July 1977, pp. 93–6, 'The Distribution of Nursing Attention in a Children's Ward', Jean Cleary, and ch. 6, published in *Nursing Times*, 7 July 1977, pp. 89–92, 'The Long-Stay Child Patient: the Problems', Roisin Pill.

Barrie Brown
Fred Clough
Jean Cleary
David Hall
Ruth Jacobs
Roisin Pill
Margaret Stacey

Foreword

Margot Jeffreys

When the editors of a volume have between them contributed to it a
lucid introduction and a forthright concluding chapter, a foreword is
likely to be otiose.

Such is the case with *Beyond Separation*. A foreword is not necessary
to draw the reader's attention to the origins of the work reported
here or to the concepts which bind the themes of the chapters
together, for this is admirably done in Chapter 1 by David Hall. Nor
do I have to point out the general and specific conclusions which
flow from the research and their relevance for the hospital care of
children, since Margaret Stacey contributes a final chapter in which
she makes specific recommendations for changes in the education
of health-service workers and in the organisation of work in wards
admitting children as well as for future research. All I can say is that
I, personally, think this book is one of the most promising to have
emerged from the burgeoning medical-sociology and social-
psychology enterprise of the last few years.

In my opinion, the authors have made out an indisputably strong
case for doctors and nurses in training to recognise that alleviating
the suffering of sick children in hospital requires the acquisition of
knowledge and skills derived from psychological and sociological
perspectives and that these are as necessary as the skills and
knowledge stemming from the laboratory-based sciences. The
former is required both to identify children most likely to suffer
psychically from the experience of hospitalisation and to alert staff
to the effects of their own behaviour on their child patients and the
latter's relatives.

The need to broaden the educational base of health workers is all
the greater because those who look after children in hospital in the
next decade are not going to have an easy time. Assuming that
public-sector expenditure on social services will be curbed in the
future, it is unlikely that resources will be forthcoming on any scale
for new hospital buildings or for substantial upgrading of present

ones. Staffing ratios are not likely to improve. Given the decline in
the birth rate, those responsible for child care will have to fight to
maintain their share of available resources against the claims of
those responsible for the care of elderly sick and multiply handicapped people, for an increasing share of those resources. Moreover,
changes taking place in the underlying assumptions about the
appropriate relationships between doctors and other health workers,
as well as between patients and health workers, can be disturbing,
especially if they are not understood.

In such circumstances, an ability to see day-to-day problems from
a more detached perspective can only help to allay dysfunctional
frustration. Research sociologists and social psychologists have been
given the task of providing that more detached perspective on the
everyday activities of human beings in small groups and in large
organisations. Their findings merit attention, and, if given it, can
help to clarify the issues with which all of us are confronted.

Of course their explanations for what they observe may, and
should be, challenged. Indeed, just as natural scientists may offer
alternative explanations for observed phenomena, so social
scientists may disagree among themselves as to the nature of the
processes they witness.

It is to be hoped, therefore, that those engaged in providing
resources and services of all kinds to children who need hospital care
will consider seriously the possible implications for their own work
of the findings of these contributions from sensitive and insightful
social scientists.

CHAPTER ONE

Introduction

David Hall

THE PILOT STUDY

In 1970 the publication of the report of the pilot study
into the welfare of children in hospital (Stacey et al.,
1970) coincided with the start of the second phase of
research at Swansea concerning children and hospitals.
The present volume contains the findings of the later
research. Although it forms a follow-up to the earlier
report, it is more than a replication of the first study.
There the major questions concerned children's vulnerability to hospital experience and several indicators were
produced which discriminated between children who were and
were not likely to be disturbed by hospital. In the present
research the problem of children's vulnerability was
still a central theme but the research progressed on a
broader base both in terms of the areas under research
and in the development of theoretical models to explain
the observations and the findings. In particular, the
research has expanded from the concern of the pilot
studies with young children in hospital for a short stay,
to consider the whole range of ages and conditions to be
found in children's wards, as well as examining the
special problems of children in long-stay wards. The
original model of the child as a social being whose
behaviour could be understood in terms of his past
experiences and what happened in the hospital has been
validated. But the emphasis has changed from a concern
solely with individual children to a consideration of the
hospital environment in equal measure and to bring out
the sociological implications of health, illness and
treatment for all concerned with children and medical
care.
    The pilot studies were undertaken between 1964 and
1967 in response to the problem that although much had

been discovered about the psychological responses of children to hospital, it seemed that a full understanding of children's vulnerability to hospital could not be achieved without an awareness of the social factors operating on the children in terms of their past experiences and learning, their socialisation into the hospital and their future development. In addition, the slowness of hospitals to adopt the reforms proposed by the Platt Report (Ministry of Health, 1959), especially unrestricted parental visiting, marked another area of concern for which a sociological explanation was required but at that time was lacking from official thinking. The desire to link aspects of individual children's responses to hospital with the analysis of behaviour as social action led directly to the multi-disciplinary approach of the pilot study, and the mixture of psychological with sociological interpretations in what was termed a 'psycho-social' approach. The same mixture of psychological and sociological research has been followed here, and while the concern with children's vulnerability to a stay in hospital has guided the direction of the research, the individual studies have selected and elaborated different themes from the basic concern with the home, the hospital, illness and treatment. The diversity that this results in is, we would argue, far from being a needless source of confusion in a topic about which some would claim enough is known already. Instead, it illustrates directly the complexity of the subject-matter. Both psychology and sociology have much to say about the health, illness and treatment of children. While we would all acknowledge a debt to the studies which first demonstrated the thesis of maternal deprivation (particularly the studies of Bowlby and the Robertsons), the theme of this volume is that just as theories of separation moved beyond a medical model of treatment of disease to show the importance of the child's attachment to his social world, so now we must move beyond separation if we are to recognise the full complexity of children's response to hospital, and having recognised the complexity, to propose and test ways of resolving the problems encountered.

THE SECOND SERIES OF STUDIES

The four projects which form the second phase of research at Swansea have a mixed origin: some were foreseen in the earlier study (Stacey et al., 1970), others added to rectify gaps in our knowledge of children in hospital.

One of the earlier studies was conducted by a psychiatrist
and a sociologist on a sample of children entering two
hospitals for tonsillectomy and adenoidectomy (op. cit.,
chs 3, 4). In addition a second sociologist conducted a
survey of parents' attitudes to, and their experiences of,
their children's treatment in hospital (op. cit., ch. 2).
The findings of these studies were summed up in a series
of practical recommendations for the amelioration of
the observed plight of children in hospital. It is from
these recommendations that there came the follow-up
study of ENT wards by Brown (1977), in the attempt to
find a convenient measure for establishing which children
were most likely to be disturbed by their hospital
experience. Also, there came the hospital playleader
research project by Hall and Cleary (1974) which sought
to investigate the effects of one particular ameliorative
measure that had been suggested.

To these projects, which arose directly from the
earlier research, two further projects were added. The
first, researched by Pill and Jacobs (1974), stemmed
from a request from the Department of Health and Social
Security for the examination of the special problems of
long-stay children in hospital. As it turned out, the
research had things to say not only about the problems
faced by the children but also about the utility of the
administrative category of 'long-stay children' in the
face of changing patterns of treatment. Second, in
accordance with the intention of developing psychological
along with sociological research, Clough's study (1975)
of two groups of older children in orthopaedic wards
brought a developmental aspect to the study of long-stay
patients.

RANGE OF THE PRESENT STUDIES

The range of studies encompassed in this volume goes
some way to meeting criticisms that have been levelled at
the earlier work, inasmuch as it had been conducted in
ENT wards and for that reason, it might be suggested,
failed to address itself to the needs of, and have more
impact on, paediatricians and those concerned with
children's wards. This criticism is, however, somewhat
misplaced, for ENT wards account for a considerable
proportion of childhood admissions and are therefore
worthy of study on that score alone; in 1972 admissions
for children under 15 to the Ear, Nose and Throat
specialty accounted for 19 per cent of all children's
admissions to hospital, making it second only to

paediatrics in terms of the number of children admitted
(DHSS and OPCS, 1974). Second, the requirements of
research design for controlling reasons for admission
and for conducting interviews and measures of children's
behaviour before admission virtually require the concentration on tonsillectomies, as the most frequent cause
of planned admissions, that was given not just in the
earlier Swansea study but in many other studies of
children in hospital. These same considerations influenced the decision of Brown to replicate the original
study in ENT wards, and it is only by relaxing some of
the stringencies of classical experimental design that
studies can be carried out in the natural setting of
children's wards. As with other aspects of the research
programme, the individual studies reinforce each other
where similar findings are made on different samples of
children, using different research methodologies.

A second criticism of the earlier studies that has
been encountered, and may be mentioned here, concerns
the representativeness of studies conducted largely in
Wales. It may be no coincidence that such criticisms
often emanated from south-east England. It is always
possible for the reader to respond to the findings of
the studies by saying that 'It doesn't happen in my
hospital' but since the publication of the earlier book,
we have been fortunate in the appearance of Hawthorn's
(1974) comparative study of nine children's wards in
south-east England, which showed that despite expectations to the contrary the quality of nursing was not far
different from that reported by Stacey et al., certainly
as far as general hospitals were concerned - and it is
in these, rather than teaching hospitals, that the
majority of sick children are nursed.

In the present studies, both Hall and Clough extended
their researches into England with the result that this
second programme of studies has not only developed on a
broader base with regard to the range of wards in which
children are nursed but also with regard to geographical
coverage. It thus provides a more substantial basis for
generalisation about the findings of specific projects.
Although hospitals differ in detail, the problems of
the provision of health care for children remain remarkably similar in different areas, which encourages us
to think of a possible convergence of theoretical perspectives and practical conclusions from the individual
studies.

THE CASE-STUDY METHOD

The method of case studies which has been used extensively
in this programme of research perhaps warrants further
comment. There is a tendency to oppose the case study
in favour of large-scale surveys and place greater
credence in generalisations derived from the latter.
But it should be clear that each method has its own
strengths and weaknesses. Cicourel (1964) contrasts the
'richness' of the former with the 'objectivity' of the
latter, but for studies of the process of patients going
through hospital, and of changes in ward environments, it
is the richness of detailed observation that is required.
   Many forms of observation were used, from Brown's
experimental situation viewed from behind a one-way
screen, through Hall and Cleary's more participant but
non-interfering ward studies, to Jacobs' living in the
orthopaedic hospital. Each project also relied upon
questionnaires as well as direct observation, and to as
great an extent as possible used a mixed strategy of data
collection. This goes some way to satisfying the requirements of Denzin (1970) for the internal validity of the
case studies. External validity, referring to the possibility of generalising research findings to other
populations, was aided by the agreement between this
research programme and the earlier Swansea studies as
well as by the replication of their studies in different
hospitals by Hall and Clough.

COLLABORATIVE INTER-DISCIPLINARY RESEARCH

Although the research programme was conceived of as a
whole, the four projects developed along largely separate
lines, while sharing some aspects of methodology and
data collection. The following chapters illustrate
different perspectives that arose out of the work, and
are designed to be read as parallel yet complementary
studies, to be brought together in the conclusion. That
this is at all possible is largely due to the emphasis
placed within the research team on co-ordination and
collaboration both in theory and practical research work.
In the course of our work we have had many difficulties,
for example, in producing a vocabulary to fit our observations that would be equally acceptable to all members of
the team. Socialisation and adaptation were particularly
difficult to translate from sociology to psychology and
vice versa, and the term discontinuity that will be
encountered in the following chapters was at best a

compromise for the processes that we thought we had seen
developing in the hospitals. In the end, I suppose, we
have to say that we define our own terms to mean what we
intend; we have not proposed a 'discontinuity theory',
but a series of interpretations around an emerging
theme which has been taken up in different ways by
different members of the team as a result of their own
observations. No general theory is intended, or is as
yet possible. However, the different perspectives
employed, which fit together round common themes, however
ill- or well-expressed they are in conceptual terms, do
go some way towards a middle-range explanation of our
observations of children in hospital.

The decision to present the research material in the
form of individual contributions rather than as a uni-
formly edited monograph is one possible approach to the
problem of reporting collaborative work. Like Jones
(1975) we have greatly benefited from regular team
meetings during the course of the work, at which
theoretical as well as methodological problems were
raised. However, a degree of independence was retained
through having the work of the sociologists and psychologists supervised by the respective departments in the
university. Unlike Jones we felt that the different
perspectives we had all brought to bear upon the question
of the welfare of children in hospital exemplified the
complexity of the research problem and that it would be
more faithful to the data, as we had interpreted them,
to present the diversity of our approach rather than
suppress it.

In an earlier article (Hall, Pill and Clough, 1976)
we attempted to sketch out the basis for thinking that
our different emphases yet contained the seeds of convergence towards a conceptual model of hospitalisation.
In that article there was space only to outline the
development of our work and thinking, and it has been
left to this volume to present the empirical data on
which our conceptualisation was based, and to draw
together the separate researches for both their theoretical
and practical content.

CHILDREN'S VULNERABILITY TO HOSPITAL: A COMPLEX PROBLEM

I think it would be fair to say that all our work
stemmed from a basic concern with the distress children
have often been observed to show in hospital, and the
deleterious consequences that have been demonstrated to
exist in many children even after their return from

hospital, in some cases persisting for months or even years. But as social scientists our concern was not simply with improving conditions (though this is important and necessary) but also with analysing the reasons why such problems should exist in organisations dedicated to the improvement of health, and why changes, when proposed, should meet with such delays as did the Platt Committee and their report of 1959 - still not completely implemented (Robinson, 1970; Hawthorn, 1974; NAWCH, 1975).

A basic message from the research is the complexity of the problem of children's vulnerability to hospital; a corollary of this is that attempts to change matters should not proceed on a simplistic model of causality - instead we need to understand the details of the relationship between a child's place in the home and in hospital in order to comprehend the significance of distress that may be exhibited (or concealed) in the wards and elsewhere. If the problem is seen as more than one of individual adjustment to a strange environment, more than separation from mother or permanent mother-substitute, it becomes relevant to enquire what effects the treatment environment has, and beyond that, what are the elements that go to constitute such an environment. The answers to these questions, we would suggest, are to be found in the nature of the interactions among the participants in the organisation of health care.

In the same way that the psychology of children's hospital experience can be broadened and improved by the addition of developmental and learning theories, so the sociology of children in hospital, which the earlier volume identified as poorly developed particularly in official governmental thinking, can usefully import perspectives developed outside hospitals, but clearly relevant to behaviour within. I am thinking of such notions as career, brought from a perspective concerned with social deviancy, and of the contribution industrial and organisational sociology has to make to the hospital as a work organisation. Some of these notions may be unfamiliar, perhaps seemingly irrelevant to those who work in hospitals and treat the children who are there. But part of the complexity that we identify has to do with the linking of the child's (and parents') perceptions of hospital and home. To concentrate on just the hospital part ignores vital elements in the problem, as the model proposed in the first study has indicated.

To summarise this argument so far, the points we wish to make that arise from the research and which have also informed the way the research has developed, are these:

(a) The psychological and sociological problems of children's disturbance in hospital are complex - certainly at least as complex as the organic problems of illness.

(b) The psycho-social cannot be reduced to a simple formula as an epiphenomenon of organic illness; hence the search for explanations that go 'beyond separation'.

(c) An explanation of children's disturbance within hospital must concentrate on both the hospital environment and that of the home, and not fragment the two.

(d) The organisational aspects of hospitals are as important for understanding individual disturbance as are the insights of psychology.

(e) The resistance to change of hospitals is not a separate problem but in part at least a further aspect of the original problem, for a system of relationships opposed to change may be related to that causing distress to children.

FINDINGS OF WIDER RELEVANCE TO THE DELIVERY OF MEDICAL CARE

From the foregoing, it should be apparent that although the major focus of research has been on children in hospital, the research cannot be limited to these topics. Indeed, I would contend that the research ultimately is not confined either to children or to hospitals. The observations, and the interpretation of the processes here offered, are applicable to other groups of special concern - the elderly, the handicapped, or patients in general, while the insights derived from hospital studies are relevant for other forms of organised care. In so far as there can be said to be one encompassing theme to our work, it lies in the delivery of medical care rather than solely in children or solely in hospitals.

The theme of medical care is illustrated in its many variations in the following chapters. Each author has been faced with the problems of interpreting his or her observations made in different hospital wards and home settings, and each has approached a solution using different sorts of interpretive models and theoretical constructs. Yet because of the sharing of an original concern with childhood vulnerability, each of the accounts is both informed by, and contributory to, the others. The reader may well find that one account is

preferable or more congenial than others; each chapter
may be treated as a separate entity - separate but
parallel. Yet all are essential and in the concluding
chapters we shall attempt some summary and evaluation of
how the different treatments of a common theme not only
express the complexity of the topic but are additive
in the theoretical model they propose and the practical
recommendations to which they point.

VULNERABILITY IN TONSILLECTOMY AND ADENOIDECTOMY

In the first of the research chapters Barrie Brown
explores the theoretical background and assumptions of
much of the earlier work on children in hospital, which
has been dominated by concerns with deprivation and
maternal separation. These concepts he interprets as
aspects of a more general balance theory, which sees
attachment behaviour in children as an evolutionary
response to threat and separation from mother. Using
this perspective he is able to review many other hospital
studies and show that although the observations of
disturbance in hospital, and in particular the phases of
disturbance reported by Robertson and Bowlby, are
explicable in terms of this model, it is less easy to
explain variations in the severity of the outcome of a
stay in hospital for different children. He concludes
that the emphasis on discontinuity which is found in
balance theory must be expanded from a purely psychological orientation to include a sociological component.
Here the meaning of discontinuity would include disruptions to the social life of the child occasioned by
hospital treatment.

In order to explore this model further, Brown's
research employed a variety of methods for investigating
home background and response to strange situations,
including hospital admission for tonsillectomy and
adenoidectomy. The methodological grounds for concentrating on this sample in the first Swansea study are still
valid, and Brown's work can be seen as a replication as
well as an elaboration of that earlier study. He
observed a total sample of forty-eight children, aged
around 5 years. The methods of research comprised experimental studies in a laboratory situation, standard psychological testing, field studies in the hospital ward and
home interviews both before and after hospital admission.

The underlying concern of the research with vulnerability was reflected in his relating of the children's
behaviour in hospital to their modes of contact with their

mothers that had been established in the home. Thus the
social organisation of the family was viewed as an
important element in the management of disturbance after
changes in the social relationships of the child on
entering hospital. Questions of maternal attitudes to
hospital experience further established the importance
of family relationships in the finding of disturbance in
children. Brown's research strongly suggests that the
biological model of mother and child has to be supplemented by an awareness of the social component in the
interactions that are fashioned and established in
families and in hospitals, and that the concept of
discontinuity may be applied not only to individual
perceptions but to the mismatch between different situations in which children find themselves.

MEANING OF ILLNESS AND TREATMENT IN ADOLESCENT ORTHOPAEDIC PATIENTS

Fred Clough, in the following chapter, also addresses
himself to the question of discrepancy of perceptions.
He is particularly concerned with the relationship between social factors of a person's background and
experiences, and outcomes in terms of observed behaviour,
through the mediation of the meanings of the situation
held by a social actor. He is also concerned with
relating psychological and sociological treatments of
discrepancy and incongruity, and in his discussion of
the meaning of illness and treatment draws a distinction
between social and personal definitions. In so far as
illness is a social phenomenon, it is structured by
expectations of social behaviour, one of the most basic
being an expectation that the sick person will seek
competent treatment. But then one is left to explain
deviant forms of illness behaviour, of failure to consult
or recourse to inappropriate remedies. In part these
may be explained by different cultural values which
operate on the illness situation in addition to the
medical model of doctor-patient interaction, but in part
they may also be affected by the personal meanings given
to illness and treatment by the sick person, who may
subscribe in general to the social norms but nevertheless
find them difficult to apply to her/his own particular
case. Fred Clough points out that the decision to seek
treatment does not necessarily imply commitment to that
treatment. While this line of reasoning is applicable
to all patients, it is particularly appropriate to those
groups of patients - the young, the elderly, the

handicapped - for whom others may exercise responsibility for their medical treatment.

The possibility of mismatch between social and personal
meanings is outlined in terms of a theory of discrepancy,
where disruption of a system of meanings lead to anomie.
In essence, it is similar to dissonance models of motivation, which link behavioural outcomes such as disturbance
with difficulties in assimilating contradictory perceptions. The problem of defining the 'standard' by which
patients evaluate their experiences is difficult and
complex. The contrast between home and hospital is
especially great, and Clough draws attention to the
importance of motivation in pursuing treatment, and the
complexity of evaluating treatment - hospitalisation, he
declares, is essentially an act of faith, where one has
to understand that staff must sometimes be cruel to be
kind. While much of the theoretical explanation of conflicts of meaning is in terms of a general model of
patienthood, Clough also shows how such an explanation
may be fitted to a development model of the information-
processing of children as presented by Piaget and others.
The conclusion is that, far from becoming unproblematic
for older children, being in hospital becomes a problem
of a different sort. While older children have the
capacity to solve some of the problems of meaning by
adopting a more sophisticated model of their situation
and in particular by adopting different time perspectives, they also acquire new sensitivities that bring
in turn new problems of dissonance to be solved or
endured.

In order to explicate the model of meanings mediating
between social background and observed behaviours, Clough
took a sample of 104 girls aged from 9 to 16 years in
the orthopaedic wards of three hospitals. Using factor
analysis, he related aspects of children's meaning
systems with staff's assessment of their behaviour to
produce an empirical classification of distinct areas of
concern identified with the home, the ward, illness and
treatment. The types of relationship predicted by the
model were found, and Clough's analysis provides a better
insight into the way in which disorders of meaning and
disorders of behaviour go together. Differences in
educational level rather than age as such were related
to differences in the organisation of meaning held by
younger and older children.

THE DENIAL OF EMOTIONS

The problem of meaning is also examined by Ruth Jacobs,
on the basis of her observations in an orthopaedic ward.
As mentioned earlier, both this research conducted by
Pill and Jacobs and that of Clough developed out of a
concern of the Department of Health and Social Security
with the special problems of long-stay children.
However, the researches have shown how these problems may
be integrated into a general model of response to hospital
experience, and how each of the separate studies illustrates different aspects of the complex interactions
between children, parents and hospital staff. Jacobs
focuses on one aspect in particular, the denial of feeling,
which she sees to be an important contribution to, as
well as a consequence of, children's disturbance in
hospital. In particular she emphasises the nature of
the orthopaedic hospital as a 'total institution' isolated
from the outside world, and discusses the consequences
for the type of control and socialisation exerted by staff
over patients. In the trend to professionalisation in
medical care, she identifies elements of depersonalisation,
of treating the patient as a work-object, and she contrasts
the treatment of illness as a matter of routine by staff
with the immediacy of illness as a crisis to the individual child (and to the parents). Her sample consisted
of thirty-eight children in an orthopaedic ward, two-
thirds of whom had congenital handicaps. Their ages
ranged from 6 months to 11 years.
   Jacobs' argument is particularly interesting in the
relation between the denial of emotion in children by
hospital staff and the estrangement of staff imposed by
the social ecology of the hospital. She shows that the
physical isolation of the hospital, possibly a historical
coincidence, appears to be related to the estranged
relationships among staff and between staff and children.
These insights, it can reasonably be suggested, are
consequential on the anthropological style of fieldwork
involving living in the hospital for several months. An
instrumental orientation on the part of the staff can
be shown to be functional to medical care, and Jacobs
categorises the mode of conflict resolution in the
hospital, where conflict was possible between hospital
staff and 'outsiders' such as teachers and parents, as
one of conflict avoidance and withdrawal. Her analysis
of time in orthopaedic hospitals is important; where
time is the healer and clinical intervention cannot speed
things up, the children are in effect 'doing time' and
given less attention by staff; in contrast, when staff

are asked for information they tend to avoid specific
references and 'play for time'. The possession of
information is related to control, and staff were con-
ceptualised as acting to reduce external threats from
children or parents. Jacobs also remarks on the discrepancy of views about the hospital episode held by staff
and by children and parents. To the staff each episode
tended to be seen as a separate incident, unrelated to
the child's past or future, which again served an instrumental and depersonalising function. The children's
viewpoint was best seen after staff had withdrawn in the
evenings, which Jacobs characterises as 'uproar'.
Otherwise there was withdrawal and depression, furthered
by staff insistence on obedience. Jacobs's analysis
relates an emphasis on meanings to sociological variables
derived from the organisation of hospitals; in doing so
she directs our attention to the nature of the hospital
as a workplace. Equally, she proposes a direct link
between studies of disturbance in children and problems
faced by staff in the pursuit of their work. In both
cases she is opening out the frame of reference from a
sole concern with children.

TASK ASSIGNMENT OR PATIENT ASSIGNMENT?

The link between the attitudes, orientations and
activities of nursing staff and the behaviour of children
in hospital is also considered by Jean Cleary. On the
basis of hospital observations undertaken during the
hospital playleader research project, she has collated
data relating to staff-patient contact from three separate
weeks of ward observation, from case studies of children
in a paediatric ward and from diary records kept by
observers. The predominant mode of organising nursing
care in the ward studied, as in most children's wards,
was through task assignment whereby a separate member
of staff performs a different item of nursing care for all,
or a batch, of children in the ward. The routine of
task assignment may be efficient for physical care but
fragments the nature of the work to the detriment of
children's social and emotional needs. While one consequence of task assignment for children is the large
number of nurses performing duties for each child, thus
increasing discontinuity of care for the child, the
consequences for nurses is also discontinuity, in that
their view of the child in hospital is fragmented. This
is in addition to the fragmentation reported by Jacobs,
where nurses treat the child in hospital in isolation from

his past and his future. History and prognosis are the
medical equivalents, but poor substitutes. Cleary's
observations about the consequences of routinisation of
work echo those of Jacobs on depersonalisation through
the application of organisational rules.

The observations reported by Jean Cleary provide
factual and quantitative data on that elusive topic of
quality of care. Particularly striking are fluctuations
in the availability of nurses during the day, not just
in the ward but in sight and earshot of the children and
potentially ready to help when requested. In common with
Jacobs she notes that the greatest amount of nursing
contact with children is made by the nurses with the
least amount of formal training. The emphasis on formal
task performance, Cleary argues, results in staff's
concentration on the task in hand to the exclusion of
other distractions - though such distractions may well
be cries for help and attention from children which if
unanswered, or unresolved, result in disturbance. Like
Jacobs, she sees conflict resolution taking place by
withdrawal and exclusion, and gives instances of the
treatment of 'difficult' child patients. The ward in
question was neither particularly below nor particularly
above average in the provision of nursing care; as far
as our different studies show, it was fairly typical of
a children's ward in a general acute hospital. The
instances that were observed in the ward were not the
result of individual lack of care but of the formal
system of care that constrained the actions of staff.
Cleary quotes other research to show that the situation
will not be remedied merely by the provision of more
nursing staff, but only by a complete re-examination of
the way in which care is provided. This chapter
provides further evidence for regarding children's
disturbance in hospital as only one feature of a complex
problem involving staff and patients in the treatment
of illness.

ILLNESS BEHAVIOUR IN A CHILDREN'S ORTHOPAEDIC WARD

The complexity of illness behaviour is a theme taken
up by Roisin Pill. She argues that health status, the
degree to which a person is capable of fulfilling valued
social roles, is as important in determining a person's
life chances as the social denominators most frequently
used, such as race, sex and social class. Thus she draws
attention to the social and cultural conditioning factors
which affect illness behaviour in medical settings.

Analysis of behaviour in hospital must be informed by
adequate knowledge of social circumstances, extending as
far back as a child's birth, and as far forward as
prognosis of the future can go. Although impairment has
a medical connotation, the definition of the term is
seen ultimately to be a social matter: it is not so much
the physical restriction that matters but the recognition
that differences in ability do exist. Pill quotes research to show that a certain range of behaviour can be
treated as 'normal', and that parents of impaired children
often treat them as normal within, and sometimes beyond,
the limitations of physical ailments.

Another useful concept dealing with children's behaviour
in hospital is that of career, which embraces both the
objective features of movement through a set of situations,
as from home to hospital to home, as well as subjectively,
the meaning attached to such movement. Pill shows how
with handicapped patients, the doctor-patient/parent
relationship differs from the 'normal' pattern usually
proposed by social scientists. Furthermore, in analysing
a study of long-stay patients made by the Welsh Hospital
Board she shows how the administrative definition of
long stay on a time basis results in a heterogenous collection of conditions, and suggests how the concept of career
could be used to generate more fruitful categorisation of
patients both for research and for administrative needs.
The relationship between patients' conditions that have
come to be defined as 'medical' or 'social' is a difficult
but important area of study, and one whose relevance is
not confined to the study of children alone.

One of the consequences of impairment, and possibly
the most important for children, is that it restricts
the socialisation of children into adult roles, not
merely in specific preparation for later life but in a
more general sense of 'learning about learning'. Using
the concept of competence, Pill argues that this demands
both empathy with other people and also the ability to
exert control over others. Handicap, therefore, has a
social effect in limiting children's opportunities to
learn, and thus restricts competence.

The validity of the concept of health status is
examined in the sample of orthopaedic patients also
studied by Jacobs. In addition Pill draws upon a series
of home interviews with children in the same sample. She
shows how the health status of children may be related
to the type of interaction children exhibit in the
hospital, and in particular to the repertoire of interactional tactics developed by children. As the role of
patient is diffuse and not specifically taught, but picked

up from interactional situations, competence in interaction is an important factor in a child being able to cope with hospital life.

SOCIAL ORGANISATION OF THE HOSPITAL WARD

Whereas Roisin Pill has demonstrated how consideration of the individual child should be extended to take into account sociological concepts of health status and social career, David Hall turns his attention to the organisation of health care, and shows how the hospital has also been a fruitful area for study and should be included in any explanation of patient behaviour. Following on from Clough and Jacobs, if we take the understanding of the meaning people attribute to behaviour as a major issue, then studies of the negotiation of interaction are particularly relevant, to direct the analysis away from a static assumption of environmental determination of action towards a dynamic perspective where social actors create the situations in which they face each other. As with Clough's model of meaning, perceptions are inserted as the intermediate link between social structures and social action. Patient role and the goals of hospitals, key elements in structural analysis, are difficult to define in detail; here it is argued there is a multiplicity of roles and goals, not explicitly pre-defined but themselves the consequences of interactional negotiations. Although the hospital remains as the locus for observations (for Hall's research concerned the introduction of playleaders into two children's wards) and although hospitals are discrete entities separated from the children's homes, they are also, as Jacobs points out, semi-permeable as organisations, and the degree to which they are 'open' or 'closed' to outside influences is itself a question for empirical research.

An emphasis on negotiations as the way in which regularities in organisations come about re-opens questions about the nature of control in organisations such as hospitals, which are not settled by reference to formal organisational principles. The patient may have an active role as participant, particularly when he may attain status as an expert in his own condition. Behaviour which from the point of view of medical professionals may be termed refusal to conform may, from the patient's view, be the assertion of his own identity and the maintenance of continuity. Power and control within the hospital is a relevant issue, and the distinction is drawn between type of control and consistency of

application, which Hall finds lacking in the wards studied;
he suggests this leads in part to children's disturbance.
    The gap between the social situation of the child in
home and in hospital is seen as one contribution to the
discontinuity of hospital stay, to the reduction of
which such solutions as play schemes may be usefully
applied. But Hall asks us to question not only the
disparity between home and hospital, but whether the
hospital situation, and even the home, do not of themselves contain elements damaging to the child. The
debate on the identification and satisfaction of children's
medical and psychological and social needs has ultimately
to be carried out beyond the sphere of the hospital,
though analysis of the hospital as an organisation can
help to put new light on the problem of children's

.TIES IN CARE

:tion has been to point the
 themes that has arisen in the
.ldren in hospital. The
 a variety of views on the
? of children in hospital,
nd that immediate theme in
rch. Each author has faced
 the data, and has drawn upon
etical perspectives, which
icern with tracing continuities
 The several authors would
ll with everything contained
 the fact that there is any
ing, the outcome of many sessions
:k and forth. What was par-
ie time was that observations
particular hospital could be
different authors in different
:o the first tentative inter-

Stacey in the final chapter
i themes that emerge, to point
; research, and from her
 director of this and the
 at Swansea into children in
:ive participant in the manage-
? practical recommendations for
.nt is not just to understand

CHAPTER TWO

Beyond Separation

Some new evidence on the impact
of brief hospitalisation on young children

Barrie Brown

INTRODUCTION

This chapter is limited in scope to a brief review of
attachment or balance theory, and a description of some
of the evidence gathered in the most recent round of
studies at University College of Swansea. Attachment
theory, perhaps because of its biological basis, has been
the most influential theoretical contribution to understanding and practice in the medical and nursing professions in relation to the plight of the young child in
hospital. The evidence described in this chapter, however, begins to suggest that there is a great deal more
than separation from mother involved in the experience
of going into hospital. This suggestion is developed and
elaborated in the subsequent chapters.

ATTACHMENT THEORY

Attachment theory derives its basic concepts from the
biological rather than social or behavioural sciences.
It draws heavily on fundamental assumptions of the etho-
logist - assumptions such as comparative continuity and
instinct. The theory has been most developed by Bowlby
(1969) and is based on the general statement that there
is a progression from simple to increasingly complex
behavioural patterns as the child ages, behavioural
patterns mediated by homeostatic control mechanisms, the
general goals of which are biological survival of the
organisms. Attachment behaviour is just such a pattern -
its specific goal is the maintenance of a certain set of
relationships between the child and mother which maximises
the probability of survival of the child. The nature of
this set of relationships is that of maintaining a close

bond between mother and child, and only those organisms
displaying the attachment system are likely to survive in
an environment containing predators. Clearly the argument
is one based on the assumption of continuity in behavioural
functions in comparative species.

Two classes of environmental events serve to elicit
attachment behaviour in the child: an enforced or
accidental disruption of the close proximity of the child
and mother, and the perception of a threat. Admitting a
child to a hospital ward without its mother can be seen
as invoking both kinds of event. The environmental
conditions that terminate attachment behaviours are the
sound, sight and tactile phenomena of the child's
mother - conditions which have led to previous attempts
to alleviate the plight of the child in hospital by the
provision of unrestricted visiting and living-in
arrangements in the hospital setting.

Attachment, however, changes as the child ages.
Indeed, both the behaviour emitted from the child and the
eliciting conditions change. As the child progresses
in age from early infancy to childhood the intensity of
overt attachment responses - crying, calling for mother,
acute distress, for example - lessens and the child
appears, perhaps superficially, to display a greater and
greater tolerance of separation and perceived threat.

Bowlby (1969) also suggests that, whilst the child
can effectively negotiate brief and limited separations
from mother, more prolonged disruption of the bond can
be most deleterious to the personality of the child
(Bowlby, 1952). Such disruptions can arise out of a
variety of circumstances, including the enforced separation of the child when admitted to hospital.

The observation that the young child may be acutely
distressed in hospital cannot be disputed. Many authors
have recorded such phenomena (for example, Edelston,
1943; Bowlby, 1952, 1960, 1961, 1968; Robertson, 1953,
1959, 1960, 1970). Bowlby and Robertson have further
proposed, however, that three sequential stages characterise the child's response during such separating and
traumatic episodes. The first phase, labelled 'protest',
can last from a few hours to a week or more. The child
cries, shakes the cot sides, throws himself about in
evident rage, and engages in repeated visual and verbose
searches for mother. At this time the child usually
proves intractable to the comforting advances of nurses,
or adults other than his mother. The next phase,
'despair', is characterised by a reduction in physical
movement, monotonous crying, and a withdrawal from any
social contact. The features of this stage have been

likened to a state of mourning. The third stage,
'detachment', is often interpreted in the practical
setting as a sign of diminution of distress, since it
usually marks a cessation of the despair phase, and an
acceptance of a nurse's attention, food and toys.
During this stage, the child is often apparently happy,
smiling and sociable with all and sundry who pass by.

Whilst there has been little controversy concerning
the observable behaviour of children during separation
in hospital, considerable debate has centered around the
attachment-theory explanation of the development of the
stages of response, and in the longer term, of the impact
of separation and deprivation derived from this explanation.

The balance-theory interpretation of the phase-
development centres around the hypothesis that the phases
are manifestations of a mourning process. Given an
instinctive tie or bond between mother and child, the
protest stage becomes an expression of chronic attachment
behaviour elicited by the inability of the child to
maintain this tie or bond in the 'normal' way. The
absence of mother, therefore, activates attachment behaviour which can never be 'switched off' whilst the mother
is absent. The second stage, despair, represents the
disorganisation which begins to permeate the attachment
behaviour when it has been chronically activated. The
effects of age on the extent of this disorganisation
are paramount, since the younger the child the less
likely it will be that re-organisation of attachment
behaviour can occur (Bowlby, 1969). In the third phase
the behavioural system of attachment becomes unconscious,
resulting in a flattening of affect which may have long-
term deleterious effects on interpersonal relationships
and the personality development of the child (Bowlby,
1952).

The attachment-theory interpretation of the child's
response to hospitalisation leads to a number of predictions which, to a greater or lesser extent, depending on
the precision of the predictions are amenable to empirical
test. Extensive reviews of the research reported in the
literature pertaining to these predictions have been
published at intervals over recent years, and the reader
is directed in particular to Yarrow (1964), Vernon et al.
(1965) and Brown (1977). It seems appropriate in this
chapter to summarise the general direction of findings
reported in this literature, and to refer the reader to
the previous reviews for more detailed criticism and
evaluation of the pertinent research.

One implication of the attachment-theory interpretation
of the child's response to hospitalisation is that the

impact of the experience will be greater in its deleterious effect the longer the period spent in the hospital and the further along the phase sequence the child progresses. Viewing in general terms the available evidence pertaining to these points, most of the empirical research confirms the progression of responses in the ward itself for all children from about 6 months to 14 years (Vernon et al., 1965).   Research into follow-up outcomes has produced far less support, however. Schaffer and Callender (1959) and Prugh et al. (1953) failed to find a relationship between duration of post-separation symptoms and length of hospital stay. It is not possible, therefore, to state that severity of outcome of the hospital experience is a function of the phase of response reached or of duration of stay.

Attachment theory would also predict that the responses of younger children would be far more overtly distressed in the hospital ward, and far more disturbed after discharge, than those of older children. Again, however, the empirical research published over the years has failed to support this prediction. Whilst some studies (see Vernon et al., 1965) have indeed found the younger child to be overtly upset, with a peak around 3 years of age, most of the research has failed to report age-related follow-up differences of the same order. One author (Douglas, 1975) has shown associations between early hospital admission (that is, repeated hospital admissions before the age of 5) and much later adolescent disturbance. This finding would seem to support the prediction derived from attachment theory that the disruption of the bond during the earlier period of its development would have a more significant and long-lasting effect than a disruption at a later age, and the author does seem prepared to suggest this causal link. Douglas goes even further, however, in suggesting much more definite causal links between precise ages of admission and precise areas of adolescent disturbance: for example, that admission during the 1-2 year period is linked to troublesome behaviour in adolescence, between 7 months and 1 year to poor reading and delinquency, and between 1 and 2 years to unstable job patterns. Apart from the criticism that can be offered concerning the import of these findings (that is, that they are in fact unique and unsupported elsewhere), there is a number of methodo-logical criticisms of the study and in particular of the suggested causal link between early admission and adolescent disturbance. Indeed, Douglas is careful to point out in the text that causal relationships between early hospital admission and later behaviour are not established by the evidence and these doubts must be reinforced. Any co-relational study contains the possibility that intervening variables between the early admission and the adolescent problem could take effect. This point has also been strongly presented in a criticism of the Douglas study by Clarke and Clarke (1976).

The writings and views of Bowlby and Robertson were most influential in the drafting of the Platt Report (Ministry of Health, 1959), particularly in recommending appropriate ameliorative facilities for children in hospital. The attachment-theory position predicts that much of the traumatic impact of the hospital experience can be offset by the frequent presence of the child's mother on the ward, if not her permanent residence there. Those studies which have examined the effects of parental visiting, however, have either failed to support the hypothesis that the presence of mother has beneficial immediate or long-term effects on the child's welfare, or have failed to provide clear evidence one way or the other (see Vernon et al., 1965). The only studies to support Bowlby (Woodward, 1959, 1962) showed that visiting does have beneficial effects on longer-term outcomes, at least for children with extensive burns, but her studies employed long-term retrospective maternal reports as the only measure of outcome and extent of visiting, and such a research design must pose considerable methodological problems.

One of the principal recommendations of the Platt Report was the advocation of facilities in children's wards for the mothers of under-5s to remain with their children throughout their stay. Both before and subsequent to Platt, many workers had published reports on mother-child inpatient units and, in general, all were impressed by the beneficial effects of such units on the concurrent and follow-up response of the child (Spence, 1946, 1947, 1951; MacCarthy, 1957; MacCarthy et al. 1962; Riley et al., 1965).

Despite such agreement only one study has tried to assess in a systematic way the concurrent and long-term consequences of a mothers-in unit. This study (Brain and Maclay, 1968) randomly assigned 197 children aged 3-6 years (having tonsillectomy) to either a mothers-in unit or a ward where visiting was restricted. All mothers were previously asked whether they wished to go in with their child if it were possible, and the children of those agreeing were included in the study.

The result of the study indicated that the mothers-in group was much better adjusted on the ward as assessed

by two ward Sisters.   The content of their assessment
seems to have been focused on frank distress, withdrawal
and interaction.

Emotional disturbance after discharge was assessed in
a psychiatric domiciliary visit by coding changes in
behaviour and physical health a few weeks and 6 months
after discharge.   The sample was classified as disturbed
if old behaviour problems and new ones were observed, and
undisturbed if there was no particular change.   Significantly more of the control group were disturbed, and
for a longer period.   Post-operative infection and
haemorrhage were more frequent in the control group.

Methodological problems, however, limit the implications for theory of this study.   Whilst theories
emphasising separation as a sufficient cause of distress
are supported by these results, the fact that the concurrent and follow-up studies were not observed blind
implies that certain biases in the results may not be
discounted.   Furthermore, would the presence of mother
have changed the nature of child-child and child-nurse
interaction in the ward sufficiently to account for the
results without recourse to separation theory?   This
possibility is in fact reflected in the statements made
by the nurses after the study had been completed: whilst
the nurses felt that having mother there curtailed any
close (i.e. mother-substitute) contact they had with the
child, her presence also significantly changed the way
they carried out physical treatments.

The aim of this brief review has been both to describe
and evaluate the ethological theory of mother-child
attachment proposed by Bowlby (1969), and to discuss its
relevance to the child's response to hospitalisation.   In
attempting to achieve this, data have been drawn from a
wide range of studies.   If conclusions can be drawn from
this mass of heterogeneous data, they can only be of the
most general kind.   Nevertheless, several points do emerge.
First, what evidence there is tends not to support the
attachment model, and therefore its usefulness must be
questioned.   Second, the nature of the theory focuses
the research worker on a series of events which occur in
a social and psychological context, but debars him from
seriously taking account of the totality of this context.
What emerges from studies in hospitals is that separation
from a single loving mother-figure, is, on its own,
neither a sufficient antecedent of longer-term psychological upset, nor distress.   Rather, where disturbance
is found, there is frequently also found the most severe
example of disruption of social experience in a more
general sense (Yarrow, 1964).   This very general

statement implies that to understand the effects of
separation a model of discontinuity must be adopted,
taking into account concepts, both at sociological and
psychological levels, which contribute to the understanding
of discontinuity. Attachment theory cannot encompass
such concepts without abandoning its inherent evolutio-
nary/ethological stance.

A STUDY OF INDIVIDUAL DIFFERENCES IN THE RESPONSE TO
A SHORT STAY IN HOSPITAL

The study reported here explores some aspects of the
notion of disruption or discontinuity in whole-family
experiences as a determinant of response to hospitalisation.
    The focus of the study is on the individual child,
aged between 3 and 6 years, admitted to hospital for
surgery, and separated from his mother and family. The
need for such a focus derives from suggestions in earlier
work, first, that only a few children exhibit manifest
signs of distress, fretfulness or disturbance during a
brief stay in hospital and second, that only a minority
of children display longer-term upset after discharge
home (Dearden, 1970). More important, however, when
the upset, or perhaps 'vulnerable', children were compared
with the rest, certain differences seemed to emerge.
The 'vulnerable' child tended to be youngest in the
family, to have a very bland or very anxious mother, to
have had less experience of meeting others, and recently
to have had an upsetting experience, such as starting
school. Differences were also isolated in terms of the
child's relationships with others; the 'vulnerable' child
found it difficult to relate to a strange adult or child,
and was generally uncommunicative.
    These tentative suggestions concerning the differences
between 'vulnerable' and other children seemed to point
to a correlation between distress in hospital on the one
hand, and certain qualities of relationships that the
child experiences in his daily life on the other. In
short, the previous findings from Swansea have suggested
that, whilst separation is an important factor in the
antecedence of upset following hospitalisation, it is
by no means a sufficient factor.
    There can be no doubt, in view of the numerous
clinical and research reports of children in hospital,
that the young child *may* be upset by a stay in hospital
without mother, even for a brief stay of a few days.
There is also agreement on the way in which the child's
response develops in stages, or phases. There is somewhat

less agreement, however, about *why* such responses should occur, or why they only occur in a *proportion* of cases (Vernon et al., 1965) and, therefore about their clinical significance when they do occur (Rutter, 1972). The lack of agreement reflects the inadequacy of explanatory devices, or models, to explain the occurrence in *some* children of upset. In the past, however, the most widely accepted model has been the balance theory of maternal deprivation (Bowlby, 1952). This model, however, leaves much unexplained, as the preceding review has shown.

The model outlined in Stacey et al. (1970) suggests that discontinuity of a more severe kind is an important determinant of the child's reaction to a hospital admission, rather than separation from mother per se. In other words, whereas the maternal-deprivation model locates the problem in a disruption of the relationship between child and mother when the child is separated in hospital, the alternative model locates the problem in a disruption of the child's social life when he is up-rooted from his family and friends and deposited in the hospital ward.

METHODS OF RESEARCH

The intention of the research was to examine the relation-ship between social processes in the family and life of the children, and variations in responses to separation and hospitalisation. The need to control for factors other than those which might influence the child's responses, for example, illness, length of stay, visiting facilities and so on, necessitated searching for a sample of young children all to experience the same surgical procedure. In this way, much more control could be gained over the factors mentioned above, and, in addition, elective surgery would give sufficient warning of admis-sion for the families concerned to be contacted and interviewed.

In a period of nine months during which cases were collected, 60 children between the ages of 3 years 0 months and 5 years 11 months were called by one hospital for T & A. Each case was passed on to the research team, giving details of name, address, age, sex and date of planned admission. Each case was first contacted by a letter to the child's mother, briefly outlining the proposed research, and requesting a preliminary interview. Of these 60 cases, 12 were lost to the research team at this stage, the reasons for loss being as follows:

4 cases cancelled admission;

2 cases were admitted too soon after notification;
5 cases were lost because mother refused to consent
to the initial interview and may or may not have
cancelled admission;
1 case was lost through default by the research team.
Examination of the sex and age distributions of the 12
lost and 48 obtained cases reveals no significant
differences.

The general research plan carried out in the project
was to collect a wide range of data from pre-admission
interviews and experimental studies, observe some of the
children in the hospital ward and then follow up as many
as possible over a period of months after discharge.
The preliminary interview was administered to all of the
sample of 48 but thereafter the sample size varied.   In
the case of the experimental and field studies, this
variation was due to the limited resources available;
only a random selection of the original sample could be
observed in the ward, 26 in all, and only 32 of the
children were taken through the experimental study.
Nineteen of the children who were observed in hospital
were also seen in the experimental aspect of the study.
The follow-up interviews were attempted for the whole
sample of 48 but some cases were lost, mainly through
bad weather, illness in the family, and holiday periods.
Only a small handful was lost through refusal by the
parents to co-operate.   This refusal rate was very small
when the demanding nature of the research programme is
taken into account.   Table 2.1 shows the demographic
details of the sub-samples in the order in which the
various aspects of the study were carried out.

First contact with the sample was at a brief initial
contact, usually by letter from myself, or by a visit
to the child's home by me.   At this meeting or contact,
a preliminary interview was arranged and this was duly
carried out.   The interviewers were all trained by myself
for this task and were instructed to use mother as the
principal informant but accepting and encouraging information from others in the family if they happened to be
present.   The first task of the interviewer was to tell
mother more about the research and then obtain her consent
to continue.   Any doubts, worries, problems and so on
were dealt with at this early stage.   The interviewer
then proceeded with a preliminary interview, structured
in two parts.   The first part was designed as a semi-
structured enquiry into the medical and social history
of the child, together with material concerning the
behaviour of the child at home and in specified situations
like starting school, being left with babysitters and so

on, data which were later used as a baseline for the follow-up assessments of post-discharge behaviour.

TABLE 2.1 Demographic details of the sub-samples used at the various stages of the research project

Time of contact	Purpose	Number	Male	Female	Mean Age*	s.d.
2 weeks before admission	Preliminary interview	48	27	21	63.27	10.00
1 week before admission	Experimental study	32**	16	16	62.00	10.16
During admission	Observation in the ward	26**	13	13	61.64	11.37
1 month after discharge	Follow-up interview	40	24	16	62.74	10.18
6 months after discharge	Follow-up interview	35	21	14	61.76	12.83

* Age, in months, at preliminary interview.
** Randomly selected cases.

The second part of the interview attempted to gather detailed information about the child's day-to-day and moment-to-moment experiences in the family. This was called the '24-hour' recall interview. It was designed to gather crude but detailed information of the minute-to-minute experience of the child at home over the previous 24 hours, as a sample of the quality of his/her family life. The 24-hour recall, based on a technique first developed by Douglas et al. (1968) for a similar analysis of the experiences of younger children, is fully described elsewhere (Brown, 1977), and the reader is referred to this work for further details of all the methodological techniques described below.

Thirty-two randomly selected subjects of the original sample of 48 were then taken in turn to the university together with their mothers, in the interviewer's car.

The aim of the experimental study was to obtain a highly detailed analysis of, first, mother-child interaction patterns, and second, the modifying effect that mother's presence and absence would have on the child's response to a brief exposure to a strange situation. The procedure consisted of placing child and mother in a small room, rather like a surgery waiting-room, containing a variety of toys. The events that occurred, the child's behaviour, and his interaction with mother, were recorded, unknown to mother or child, on a videotape machine hidden behind a one-way screen. A few minutes later, a stranger entered the room, sat down, and appeared to take notes, then a little while later, mother was asked by the stranger to leave, and later still, the stranger also left, leaving the child now quite alone. At this point if the child was distressed the mother was called back into the room, but if frank distress did not occur, mother only came back after several minutes. The recordings were so arranged that they could be divided into sequential 5-second units, and in the subsequent analysis the events that took place in each of the situations could be described in terms of the frequency of occurrence of certain categories of behaviour, such as talking to mother, picking up and fingering or playing with a toy, and so on. A similar analysis is reported by Kalverboer (1971).

When the experiment was completed, the mother was asked to fill in a series of questionnaires concerned with her attitudes to rearing and the child's hospitalisation. Meanwhile, the child was asked to complete the Bene Anthony Family Relations Test (Bene and Anthony, 1957).

Twenty-six of the original 48 children were randomly selected for observation in the hospital ward. Nineteen of these 26 were also seen in the experimental situation. Observation in the ward was carried out by personnel trained by myself, employing a mixed time-and-activity sampling technique similar to that employed by Pill (1967). Observations were made throughout the child's waking periods from the moment of admission to the fifth day. Most children were discharged on the sixth day.

All 48 mothers were contacted again 1 month and 6 months after the child's discharge from the hospital, when a semi-structured interview designed to assess changes in the child's medical and behavioural state was administered. The opportunity was also taken to check on major changes in the circumstances of the family and child.

THE CHILD IN THE HOSPITAL WARD

The ward into which the children were admitted was of the
corridor variety, having a long window-flanked corridor
with a series of cubicles on one side with each cubicle
containing two or three beds. Amenity, treatment and
Sister's rooms were in the centre of the block, with
toilet and playroom facilities at one end and an adult
toilet and linen closet at the other. An operating
theatre was attached to the ward with direct access into
the main corridor, in a position opposite the Sister's
room. This layout enabled observers to watch the
children with a minimum of interference, either with
on-going ward activity or with the activities of the
children. The observers sat in the corridor opposite
the open door of the cubicle and were thus able not only
to see and hear what happened in the cubicle but also to
know where the child had gone if the child left it.
The observers recorded events from the moment of admission
to the ward to the end of the fifth day, noting down on
a record sheet what happened to the child from minute to
minute, what the child said and to whom. In practice,
these recordings were made from 8.00 a.m. to 8.00 p.m.
In addition, blood pressure and temperature readings
were collected every day from the ward records.

The end result of all this observation was a detailed
record of the child's stay. The data obtained were
subjected to a principal-components analysis: in other
words, all the records for all the children were compared
and the main dimensions of response extracted. The
emphasis in this analysis, therefore, was to describe
how the sample as a whole varied in its response to the
hospital: the dimensions, three in number, are a convenient way of describing simply how this variation
occurred. The emphasis was not to isolate individual
children who were particularly upset.

The analysis revealed that the sample's response to
the ward could be described in terms of three dimensions
or tendencies: 'withdrawal', 'immobility' and 'distress'.
The withdrawal dimension refers to the extent to which
the children became involved in interactions with others:
children who scored high on this dimension tended to keep
away from others, talk very little to parents, children
or staff, not become involved in games with other
children. In contrast, children who scored low on this
dimension were very talkative, very interactive, playing,
talking and becoming involved not only with parents but
with other children, other visitors and staff.

The second dimension was called immobility because it

refers to the tendency to stay within the cubicle area. Children who scored high on this dimension rarely moved out into the corridor or to the playroom, spent a long time in or on their beds and rarely moved about the ward. Children who scored low were very much more mobile around the ward, spending time in other cubicles, in the playroom and along the corridor.

The third dimension was called distress because it referred to the tendency with which the child showed frank upset and physiological disturbance. Children who scored high on distress cried, screamed and grimaced a great deal, rarely smiled or laughed, tended to stay close to parents when they visited, and showed marked increases in blood pressure and temperature towards the end of their stay in the ward. In contrast, children who scored low were much less upset, laughed more, were less clinging to parents when they visited, and showed steady declines in blood pressure and temperature throughout their stay.

In describing these dimensions of response, a distinction must be made between this kind of analysis, which describes the responses of the sample as a group rather than describes the responses of individual children, and the kind of analysis which divides the group up into sub-groups of individual children based on response tendencies. Whilst the latter kind of analysis was not used here, it is possible to take a few children from the sample and show how the dimensions of response can be used to describe the individual child.

THREE EXAMPLES

Child 1

Male, aged 5 years 6 months at first interview, second oldest of three children, having been at school for 1½ years, with mother not at work and father an unskilled factory worker. On arrival at 2.00 p.m. on the first day he spends the first two hours out of bed but does not wander far from the cubicle. Mother stays with him until the early evening and he talks to her and the other child in the cubicle from time to time. For more than half the time he sits near the bed doing nothing at all. After mother leaves he cries for a moment or so, then settles into bed. On the second day, he is given pre-medication in the morning, and stays in bed until wheeled into the theatre just before midday. He is asleep then until the early evening, about 6.00 p.m. when he takes a little nourishment and talks to his parents for a few moments. On the third day he stays in his cubicle nearly all day, lying in bed in the morning and playing in the afternoon. He is a little fretful during the morning when mother is there but cheers up in the afternoon. Although mother talks to him a great deal he does not reply very much, but, when mother goes away during the lunch period, he talks for a while to the other child in the cubicle. Most of his interaction with others during the day, in fact, consists of playing games with this other child. When his parents leave again in the evening he cries again for a moment but settles down very quickly, and goes to sleep a few minutes later. On the fourth and fifth days he is much more mobile, spending most of the day out of his own cubicle. Mother and father again visit for much of the day but although they talk to him a lot and cuddle him he rarely talks back. Most of his interaction is with the other children, and takes the form of play without verbal interactions. On these days he cries a little during the day but there are no more tears when mother leaves. In the analysis he scores high for withdrawal, fairly low for immobility and about average for distress.

Child 2

Female, nearly 6 years old at first interview and second oldest of three children but with a much older step-brother of her father's first marriage. She has been full time in school for more than a year, mother does not go out to work and father is a clerk in local govern-ment. This little girl scores very low for withdrawal but average for distress and immobility. On the first day she is fairly active after admission, moving around the ward exploring, talking at great length with the other children and nursing staff. Mother leaves fairly soon after midday, having spent just the first hour with her, and she cries for a while after she has gone. For the rest of the day, though, she seems quite settled and even strikes up a humorous conversation with another child's mother. She goes for operation on the next day just before midday but spends the earlier part of the morning playing and talking with the children in the next cubicle. After the operation she sleeps for the rest of the day. On the third, fourth and fifth days she is much less mobile but remains remarkably talkative with everyone and not at all distressed, except for the morning after the operation when she is still very tired.

Child 3

Male, aged 5 years 5 months at first interview and the
elder of two children. Had started school at 4½ years,
mother not working and father a farm worker in a remote
valley to the north. This child scored average for
withdrawal and immobility but very low on distress.
Indeed, the remarkable characteristic about this child
was the fact that he spent so much of his time laughing.
Throughout his stay he played, talked and moved around
the ward to a moderate degree, was not upset prior to
the operation and never once cried when mother and father
left for home. His interaction with others was spasmodic
but was always characterised by joking, laughter and fun.

These three examples show how the three dimensions of
response to hospital can be translated into individual
responses and, incidentally, demonstrate how any individual
child can be a high scorer on one of the dimensions of
response but a low scorer on the others. Throughout
the subsequent discussion, the dimensions of response
of the sample will be used, the data thus not referring
to individual children's responses.

HOME EXPERIENCE AND HOSPITAL RESPONSE

The 24-hour recall interview was designed to give a
measure of the quality of the child's life at home, and
the protocols gathered from the home interviews were
analysed using the same sort of analysis as for the
hospital responses. This analysis revealed that the
home experiences of the children could be simply described
again in terms of three dimensions: 'initiation',
'subordination' and 'proximity'. These terms, it must
be emphasised, are simply arbitrary labels for empirical
dimensions emerging from the analysis. The terms were
chosen because they seem to describe best the content of
each dimension. Initiation refers to the extent to which
the child in the family seems to have some control over her/
his own activities. Children who scored high on initiation were likely to be rather more in control of what
they did, who they interacted with, for how long and
when. In contrast, children who scored low on initiation
tended to exert such control to a lesser extent. The
second dimension, subordination, refers to the extent to
which families extend control over the child in her/his
day-to-day activities. Children who score high on this
dimension tend to have their activities determined by

others and, in addition, tend to spend more time outside the home, excluding time spent at school. Moreover, they seem to stay close, though not in physical contact, when they are at home. Children who score low on this dimension are much less controlled, spend less time outside the home but do not necessarily stay close to other family members. The third dimension, proximity, refers to the extent to which the child seems to be involved or integrated into family activities. The children who score high on this dimension spend a lot of time in the house, tend to spend a lot of time in close proximity to other people and watch television a great deal. Children who score low on this dimension are outside much more, are often separated to a high degree from other family members and spend less time watching television.

Significant correlations between hospital response and home experience were computed. It was found that children who scored high for family proximity tended also to score very high for distress in the hospital. Children who scored high for initiation at home, on the other hand, were very little distressed in the hospital but were also very mobile and interactive, scoring low on both immobility and withdrawal. However, the highly proximate child at home was also very mobile in the hospital. In other words, there is a tendency for the distressed child in hospital to come from a family in which he is a low initiator and very high on proximity. The immobile child, in contrast, although also a low initiator comes from a low-proximity family. The withdrawn child in the hospital tends to be a low initiator at home. Table 2.2 shows the correlation coefficients between the three hospital-response measures and the three family-experience measures, demonstrating these relationships.

CHILDREN'S RESPONSE AND FAMILY COMPOSITION

One explanation of the relationship between hospital responses and family experiences could be the effect of the size of the family. Many studies have suggested that children from large families have poor verbal intellectual development when compared with children from small families (for example, see Rutter and Mittler, 1972) and the possibility has been raised that this difference can be accounted for by the quality of family life in preference to genetic differences. Bossard and Boll (1960) have shown that families of different sizes do indeed create different types of interaction patterns

TABLE 2.2   The relationship between hospital response and family experiences in a sample of 26 children

Hospital response	Family-experience dimensions		
	Proximity	Subordination	Initiation
Distress	+0.699**	—0.303	—0.597**
Immobility	—0.559**	—0.280	—0.459*
Withdrawal	+0.260	+0.003	—0.869**

Pearson product moment correlations
*   significant p < 0.05
** significant p < 0.01

at home, as well as sharing different value and belief systems. Since the foregoing evidence points to a relationship between hospital response and family experience, the question has to be asked: Can these differences be linked to size of family?

In the present study, however, family size was apparently unrelated to hospital responses on the ward. Although the range of family sizes was small in the sample, the biggest being 6 children, by comparing children from families with 4 or more children with those from families with 2 or 3 children, and with only children, no significant differences between size and hospital response could be found. Table 2.3 shows the results of the Kruskall-Wallis one-way analysis of variance test on these data.

TABLE 2.3   The relationship between family size and response in the hospital

Hospital response	Kruskall-Wallis H	p
Distress	0.838	NS
Immobility	1.020	NS
Withdrawal	0.281	NS

Another aspect of family composition, however, is the ordinal position of the child in the family group of children. Dearden (1970) suggested in her study of post-hospital adjustment that the only and youngest child might experience greater difficulties after a hospital stay, a point which is emphasised for practical reasons in the discussion of her study by Stacey (Stacey et al., 1970). When ordinal position was examined in this study, however, there were tendencies for only children to be *less* distressed in the ward, although the youngest children showed a slight tendency to be more withdrawn. Comparison of these two findings is made difficult because of the problems of comparing responses in the ward with those after discharge.

PREPARATION FOR ADMISSION

The Platt Report (Ministry of Health, 1959) makes the recommendation that it is the parents who should be encouraged to prepare the child for elective admission, bearing in mind the age and peculiar needs of the individual child. However, there are two perhaps related issues at stake here: first, different families might, for a variety of reasons, be capable of preparing their child with different degrees of efficiency. Second, families might have doubts whether they ought to provide preparation at all, and, more subtly, will have very definite ideas about what sort of preparation to give, based perhaps on many factors, including what their relatives and neighbours thought and did. In short, how the child is prepared for an elective admission may well be best left to parents but there is no guarantee that the individual parent will either know how, or indeed be prepared, to carry out the task.

The mothers were asked, about two weeks prior to the child's admission, how they had prepared, or would prepare, their child. The interviewers were instructed to give no hint of what might or ought be said, although by the time of the interview every mother had received a copy of the hospital information booklist, which contained a list of useful hints about what to bring, visiting and so on.

Mother's comments about what she had said or would say to the child were recorded by the interviewer and later classified into eleven categories. Table 2.4 shows these eleven categories, together with the number of mothers mentioning each. The total adds up to more than 26 because many mothers mentioned more than one. Most mothers reported up to two or three separate items. The most common items of preparation were information about what was to happen, category 3, which incidentally was rarely explained in anything but the vaguest detail, and there being toys and other children to play with, category 6.

TABLE 2.4 Categories of information and the number of mentions by mothers as given to their children

Category	Content	Number of mentions
1	No information	0*
2	Nice things to eat, ice cream and jelly	8
3	Tonsils cut out	14
4	Put to sleep with injection	5
5	Be in hospital for several days	4
6	Toys and other kids to play with	9
7	Make better	1
8	Make throat/ears better	5
9	Nurses/doctors nice	3
10	Look at throat	1
11	Child will stay without mother	2
		$\overline{52}$**

* One mother of a child not observed in the ward said she had told her little girl that she was going on a short holiday.
** Average per mother = 2.

In order to assess the effect of different qualities of preparation in children, some way had to be found of dividing the sample of children into groups according to different qualities of preparation received. In the literature, there are two main themes in relation to preparation: one theme suggests that information relieves the child from distress because it gives the child foreknowledge and hence some expectation of medical procedures and, in addition, counteracts the sometimes dramatic and false rumours that surround hospital experiences for children in the classroom and playroom (Vernon et al., 1965). Other themes include the need to express emotional tension as a cathartic exercise and the need to develop trust and confidence in staff; but perhaps the most important is the distinction between factual information as a preparation and information which essentially reassures the child. Accordingly, the eleven categories of information were divided into two groups: information, numbers 3, 4, 5, 7, 8, 10 and 11; reassurance, numbers 2, 6 and 9. The distinction between the two types of information is, primarily, that factual information is seen as confronting the child with reality, whereas reassurance, whilst not actually presenting false information, essentially attempts to buffer the child against the possibility of unpleasantness by focusing on the nice things that are to happen.

The children could now be divided into three groups: those who received only information (7 children), those who only received reassurance (6 children) and those who received a mixture of both (13 children). These three groups were then compared in their responses to the ward, a comparison which showed that the only significant difference to arise was that children who were given only factual information were much more mobile around the ward than children who were given reassurance only. In other words, the quality of preparation seemed to make very little difference to the child's response in the ward except for this single effect. Table 2.5 shows the results of the Kruskall-Wallis tests, to demonstrate this point

TABLE 2.5 Comparison of preparation qualities in hospital response

Hospital response	Kruskall-Wallis H	p
Distress	0.772	NS
Immobility	5.919	0.05*
Withdrawal	2.073	NS

* Mann-Whitney U-tests of the group difference shows that those receiving information are significantly less immobile than those receiving reassurance only.

There is now a considerable body of evidence (reviewed in Vernon et al., 1965) which suggests that when it is known that the child has been factually prepared, benefit does result in follow up and sometimes during admission itself. In this sample, any effect of the differences in preparation quality is probably hidden by an overall paucity of the information, and possibly by the arbitrary nature of the definitions of reassurance and information.

CHILDREN'S RESPONSE AND MATERNAL ATTITUDES

The pilot study (Stacey et al., 1970) had reported that there was a tendency for children with either highly anxious or non-anxious mothers to show up as abnormal on the global measures of follow-up response. Some authors, indeed, have theorised that parental anxiety may adversely affect the child's reactions to hospital experiences, perhaps through some process of social contagion. Such a hypothesis is suggested by the findings of Campbell (1957) with respect to infants' reactions to inoculations and in the post-hospital studies of Weinick (1958) and Woodward (1959), but in none of these studies is it suggested that very low anxiety may also relate to adverse responses.

In the present study, several aspects of mother's anxieties about hospitalisation, her anxiety about her child, acceptance of authority, attitudes to the ability of the hospital to care for her child and visiting, were assessed in 19 out of the 26 cases. These 19 cases were randomly selected from the whole sample of 48, since they are those cases that were involved in both the hospital observations and the experimental study. The assessments were carried out by using the questionnaire format developed by Robinson (1967), based on the method devised by Shapiro (1961), and categorised the mothers on each attitude as high, medium or low.

TABLE 2.6   Distribution of 19 mothers on the five attitude scales

Attitude scales	High	Medium	Low
Anxiety about own hospitalisation	2	7	10
Acceptance of hospital authority	10	4	5
General anxiety about the child	4	5	10
Acceptance of hospital's ability to care for child	15	3	1
Need for mother to visit child in hospital	17	2	0

Table 2.6 shows that there is little variance in the sample in attitudes to visiting and care of children in

hospital, a finding which replicates that of Robinson (1967) using the same instrument. The remaining three scales, however, discriminate much better amongst the sample, and Table 2.7 shows the relationship between each of these three scales and the three hospital-response dimensions.

TABLE 2.7 The relationship between child's hospital response and maternal attitudes, in 19 cases

Attitude scale	Child's hospital response		
	Distress	Immobility	Withdrawal
Acceptance of hospital authority	H = 13.86*	H = 1.352	H = 0.572
Anxiety about child	H = 0.980	H = 16.87*	H = 0.390
Anxiety about hospitalisation	H = 0.976	H = 0.939	H = 21.015*

All tests refer to Kruskall-Wallis one-way analysis of variance.
* $p < 0.05$.

Table 2.7 shows three significant relationships and Mann-Whitney U-tests show that these three relationships resolve themselves as follows: mothers who are highly accepting of hospital authority have children who are highly distressed; mothers who express general anxiety about their children tend to have children who are immobile in the hospital; mothers who are themselves anxious about hospitalisation tend to have children who are withdrawn in the hospital.

These findings generally reflect on what has been suggested in the literature for many years: that children are extremely sensitive to the feelings and attitudes of those in close contact with them (Bowlby, 1960; Coleman, 1950), a suggestion which has clear implications in this field. Robinson (1967) has suggested that mothers pass on their fear about hospitalisation through non-verbal clues and through behaviour which avoids the fear situation, resulting in highly anxious mothers spending less time in preparing their children, and perhaps less time in taking advantage of unrestricted visiting and living-in facilities.

The evidence on preparation does not seem to support

this conjecture in the present study, since, despite the clear relationships between attitudes and hospital responses, differences in preparation seem to be largely unrelated to what happens in the hospital. The present analysis does not allow causal explanations to be derived from the data, but the implied relationships emerging from a comparison of Tables 2.2 and 2.7 lead to the tentative conclusion that certain types of maternal attitude may have roots in certain types of family environments. Such a conclusion reinforces the tentative implications put forward by Robinson that more attention could profitably be focused on the *parents* when the welfare of their *children* in hospital is being considered. Furthermore, it suggests that such attention should not only involve parental attitudes but also broader influences on the child.

CHILDREN'S RESPONSE AND VISITING

If highly anxious mothers tend to avoid the fear-invoking situation - the hospital - and by so doing contribute to the discontinuous nature of the transition from home to hospital, it might be expected that amount of visiting by mother will relate to the child's response to hospital, although, of course, many factors other than her fear of hospital will contribute to her actual visiting behaviour. In this study, mothers were asked in the follow-up interviews how much time was spent visiting, both by themselves and other members of the family. The answers received suggested that mothers spent from about 20 to 48 hours on the ward out of a possible total of about 72 hours, and that about the same amount of time was spent on the ward by other visitors. Table 2.8 shows the Pearson product moment correlations between the number of hours of visiting by mother and others and the three hospital-response dimensions.

One interpretation of the results shown in Table 2.8 is that the effect of mother's visiting on hospital responses was limited to restricting the mobility of the child (perhaps by encouraging the child to stay close to mother while she was there). Visiting by mother or others appears to play no part in affecting distress or withdrawal. The data in Table 2.8 are not to be taken to mean, however, that visiting does little to alleviate the child's problems when in the hospital. The actual number of hours mother spends in the ward is much less important than what she does, or is allowed to do, when she is there.

TABLE 2.8 Coefficients of correlation between visiting and hospital response

	Distress	Immobility	Withdrawal
Time spent in hospital by mother*	−0.142	+0.525***	−0.160
Time spent in hospital by all visitors**	+0.014	+0.308	−0.041

*   Hours visited by mother: mean = 32.40 hours; standard deviation = 8.19 hours.
**   Total hours visited: mean = 56.00 hours; standard deviation = 12.62 hours.
*** $p < 0.01$.

THE LABORATORY STUDY OF MOTHER-CHILD INTERACTION

The data pertaining to the children in the hospital ward have shown that differences in response can be related to differences both in family experiences, and in mother's attitudes to the hospital and her anxiety about hospitalisation. These relationships seem to predominate over other possible correlates of hospital response such as visiting, preparation, family size and ordinal position.

A concept which might explain the relationship between family experiences and hospital response is continuity of care of the child, a concept which emphasises not so much the separation of the child from her/his mother, as the break in relationships with members of the family imposed by the move to hospital. It has been suggested, further, that the impact of this break in continuity is greater for some children than others, depending on the characteristics of the relationships that they have at home. The family-experience dimension strongly suggests that the break is worse for the child who comes from a close-knit family structure, who is unused to initiating relationships with others. Such a child is likely to be very distressed and withdrawn in the hospital ward. The purpose of the laboratory studies was to show that a concept like 'proximity' could be studied in detail under controlled conditions, perhaps leading to some suggestions about the mechanisms which might mediate between particular types of family experience and particular types of response to the hospital.

An experimental study was carried out on 32 of the original sample of 48, and 19 of these 32 were also observed in the hospital ward. The procedure adopted resembled closely the study published by Ainsworth (1969) of the interaction between infants and mothers in a strange situation. One aspect of the laboratory study was an examination of the strategy adopted by the child in maintaining contact with mother under novel conditions. The 32 children taking part were closely observed and were categorised according to the degree to which visual and verbal modes of maintaining contact with mother were adopted.

Results from this study suggested that contact styles were related to the exploratory behaviour of the children when separated from mother. Children who employed high rates of visual contact were found to show a significant decline in exploration when mother left the room. At the same time, these children also showed a massive increase in distress.

Contact styles were also found to relate to the three family-experience dimensions - high visual contact being positively related to proximity, and high verbal contact to low subordination. Children who engaged in high rates of visual contact with mother were much more likely to have expressed protest or distress when left with someone else, although the frequency and incidence of being separated from mother was no different. High visual contact was also found to occur in children whose mothers were much more likely to accept hospital authority, and were much more anxious about the child.

These data may suggest a way of explaining the individual child's attempts to deal with novel and separating situations like the hospital ward. The explanation is tentative but can be gleaned from several independent sources. What typifies the high-proximity and non-initiating child is a reliance on visual contact with mother, at the expense of verbal contact or self reliance; children who indulge predominantly in visual contact are also likely to display distress in a range of situations which involve separation and the imposition of novelty - starting school, being left with babysitters and so on. Taken together, this evidence might be seen as support for the notion that the act of separating mother and child is not a sufficient condition for psychological upset. Rather, given that the conditions of the separation are the same for all in terms of length of stay, opportunity for visiting and so on, severe problems will arise when separation occurs in a family context which is of a particular quality, a quality which emphasises the need for family members to be physically close to each other.

PROBLEMS AFTER DISCHARGE

There has been a number of attempts to describe and
account for children's psychological responses to a stay
in hospital, but few attempts to carry out systematic
analysis of responses in the long term after discharge.
Two such studies, however, have been reported in the
literature: Vernon et al.(1966) attempted to evaluate
changes in 387 children by means of a retrospective
questionnaire sent through the post to each child's
mother just one week after the child had been discharged
from hospital. Pill (1974) used the same questionnaire,
administered in person to the mothers of a sample of 39
children admitted to an orthopaedic ward. These, and
other less systematic enquiries, have concentrated on
variations in the hospital experience - usually length
of stay, amount of visiting, age when admitted, and
preparation for admission - and neglected such child
variables as pre-hospital adjustment (except for Jessner
et al., 1952), and in particular the child's relationship
with others. The purpose of this section is to show how
follow-up responses relate to such variables, and, in
addition, to assess the relationship between response to
hospital and follow-up responses. The samples used in
the two follow-ups, at one month and six months after
discharge, are described in an earlier section.

The assessment used by Vernon et al. (1966) required
mother to assess behavioural changes in her child retrospectively, just one week after the child's return home.
The employment of a postal questionnaire resulted in many
mothers not replying. In the present study both these
problems are circumvented by face-to-face questioning and
by avoiding the need for a pre-post hospital comparison.
This was achieved by interviewing mother before admission,
then twice afterwards, and on each occasion asking her
to describe her child's behaviour at that time.

A factor analysis of Vernon's questionnaire revealed
six main types of response: general anxiety, separation
anxiety, sleep anxiety, eating disturbance, aggression
and apathy. The present study employed these six factors
plus a rating of general health, but without using the
precise format of the questionnaire. Mother was questioned
in a fairly unstructured way on each of the three
occasions, the discussion focusing on the same areas of
behaviour on each occasion. Coders then examined the
protocols and rated each child for each of the factors
as 1 for improved, 2 for no change, or 3 for worse, by
comparing the first interview with the second and third
respectively. In order to avoid interviewer bias, the

same interviewer was never used for more than one of
the three interviews. Table 2.9 shows the results of
these interviews.

TABLE 2.9   Changes in behaviour* in the sample at one
month and six months after discharge from hospital

Factor	Better		Same		Worse	
	1m	6m	1m	6m	1m	6m
General health	72	88	20	3	8	9
General anxiety	35	51	30	26	35	23
Separation anxiety	28	57	32	23	40	20
Apathy	15	26	85	74	0	0
Aggression	18	23	52	62	30	15
Sleep anxiety	30	57	38	23	32	20
Eating disturbance	30	62	70	38	0	0

* Figures shown are percentages of total sample (40 at
1 month, 35 at 6 months).

   For the three anxiety factors, approximately one third
of the children are placed in each category after one
month, but by six months more than half are in the
'better' category. For general health, only a few
children did not show improvement even at one month.
For apathy, little change was recorded at either follow-
up. For aggression more than half of the children show
no change, for eating disturbance no children show a
worsening, and most show improvement by six months.
   There is some disagreement in the views expressed in
the literature on the incidence of problems after discharge
from hospital, some suggesting that most children recover
quickly, but others (Jessner et al., 1952) pointing to a
degree of upset in the majority of cases for some months
after discharge. The data presented in Table 2.9 suggest
that there are few problems in general health, and
eating has improved as a result of the tonsillectomy and
adenoidectomy operation, even at one month, a finding
that fits well with the previous evidence on the effects
of such operations on young children. By six months,
moreover, for most factors there are more children in
the improved category than elsewhere, a finding which
would seem to suggest that the incidence of behavioural
problems over the long term is not very high for children

of this age having this operation. The Jessner et al.
study, also of young children having ENT surgery, however,
presented clinical evidence to the effect that a majority
of children has at least some behavioural disorder on
follow-up. Table 2.10, therefore, shows how many children
displayed any problems at the two follow-ups and suggests
that whilst few children showed more than two problems,
even at six months less than half the sample were showing
none.

TABLE 2.10 Incidence of any 'worse' ratings in the sample
one month and six months after discharge

Number of worse ratings	0	1	2	3+
1 month	7	13	16	4
6 months	15	12	6	2

Chi square = 19.486.
df = 3.
p < 0.001.

Nevertheless, there is a significant move towards fewer
problems, a finding which supports the report by Dearden
(1970) using global scores of psychological adjustment.

THE RELATIONSHIP BETWEEN HOSPITAL RESPONSES AND FOLLOW-UP
RESPONSES

Bowlby (1969) has argued that the child who is distressed
and overtly disturbed by the hospital-ward situation is
showing a normal reaction to separation from mother and that
the same child should have a good chance of recovering
quickly once a 'satisfactory' relationship with mother
is re-established at home, with limitations imposed by
the age of the child and the extent of trauma associated
with the hospitalisation. In contrast, Bowlby argues,
the child who shows no distress when in hospital is
likely to exhibit some disturbance on return home, since
the display of calmness and adjustment in the hospital is
evidence of some abnormality of mother-child relationship.
Is it the case in the present study that the child who
is upset in the hospital is likely to show fewer
behavioural problems after discharge?
    Of the 26 children observed in the hospital, 22 were
followed up at one month and 19 at six months. Table 2.11
shows the relationship between the ratings of behaviour
after discharge and the child's response to the ward itself.

TABLE 2.11 The relationship between behavioural response during follow-up and response to the ward*

Response to the ward	General anxiety		Separation anxiety		Sleep anxiety	
	1m	6m	1m	6m	1m	6m
Distress	16***	27**	55	53	45	22***
Immobility	53	22**	34	27**	43	40
Withdrawal	48	54	35	29	33	27***

	Aggression		Apathy		Rating		General	
	1m	6m	1m	6m	1m	6m	1m	6m
Distress								
Immobility			No significant relationships					
Withdrawal								

*   Figures are U-values from Mann-Whitney U-tests of ranked hospital-response scores for 'better' compared with 'worse' and 'no change' categories combined.
**   0.05 $p < 0.10$
*** 0.01 $p < 0.05$.

None of the relationships is very marked but there is a trend for lack of improvement in general anxiety to relate to high distress and high mobility. Children who show no improvement in separation anxiety at one month tend to be less withdrawn in hospital, but lack of improvement in separation anxiety at six months relates to more withdrawal in hospital. Sleep anxiety is more closely related to distress and withdrawal in hospital only at six months. None of the other behavioural ratings bears any relationship to hospital response, neither is there any clear relationship between number of problems and hospital responses.

In short the link between hospital responses and follow-up responses is at best a confused and rather weak one. Whilst there is some evidence of distress in hospital being associated with general anxiety and sleep anxiety after discharge, withdrawal seems to bear a very mixed relationship to what follows. Immobility, on the other hand, seems to relate to less separation anxiety initially and less general anxiety in the long run. There does, however, seem to be little evidence of the inverse relationship between hospital disturbance and follow-up disturbance, as proposed by Bowlby (1969).

PREDICTING DISTURBANCE IN THE HOSPITAL

The general theme of the study thus far is towards the
identification of family-experience dimensions that appear
to relate to different responses to hospital. The discussion has isolated the high proximity and non-initiating
child as particularly at risk. Some of the additional
features of the at-risk child, features that can be seen
as consistent with those family experience characteristics,
are the presence of other siblings with whom there is
likely to be competition, an anxious mother, and a dependence on simple visual strategies of interaction with
other people. In this section an attempt is made to
elicit directly from the child data which seem to relate
to these family characteristics. For a number of reasons
it was not possible to carry out these procedures with
the whole sample, and the data available refer only to
those children assessed in the laboratory situation.
However, since the laboratory study was able to show that
predominantly visual-contact styles with mother were
closely related to distress in hospital, there seems to be
some justification for attempting to identify the high
visual-contact children as an indirect means of detecting
children at risk.
     In this section, therefore, an attempt is made to
establish a relationship between what was observed to
occur when the child and mother were together in the
strange situation and what the child feels and thinks
about relationships with others at home. This might
suggest how 'at-risk' children (that is children who are
likely to respond to a separating and strange experience
with overt upset and perhaps longer-term disturbance)
might be quickly, and reliably, detected in practical
situations - the outpatient clinic prior to admission for
surgery for example.
     The technique employed to describe the child's view
of his family dynamics is the Bene-Anthony family-relations
test (Bene and Anthony, 1957). This test has been widely
used in clinical practice in this country as a technique
for eliciting the child's view of the structure of
relationships within the family group. The FRT essentially
dramatises the child's perception of his family, rendering
its administration both popular with, and easy for,
children of all ages from about 5 years upwards.
     The FRT consists of line drawings of men, women, boys,
girls and babies, each having minimal features. To each
of these is assigned a red postbox. The test is presented
to the child as a postman game and figures are chosen
from a pool by the child to represent members of his

family. Statements like 'This person in the family likes me' are posted by the child to the member of the family for whom (for the child) the statement is true. An additional figure, 'Mr Nobody', is introduced by the psychologist, to whom all statements not belonging to anyone in the family are posted. In the junior version of the test there are 40 statements divided into five groups of 8. Each group defines a notional type of state-ment, like 'outgoing positive', and the grouping of statements is used, by those employing the test as a diagnostic aid, as the framework for scoring the test.

Thirty-two of the children (the same sample admitted to the laboratory study) were administered the junior version of the FRT about two weeks prior to admission. The tests were carried out in a university building as part of an extensive battery and, although mothers were near at hand, they were not involved in this part of the programme.

The analysis of the FRT data was designed to answer two questions. First (see Figure 2.1B) the distribution of the items in the test (that is, assignment of items to self, mother, father etc.), was calculated for the 'at-risk' children (that is, the 6 children who employed a very high rate of visual contact with mother in the experimental situation) and for the remaining 26 of the sample (Figure 2.1C). This first analysis shows that the 'at-risk' children are more likely than the rest to assign items to siblings but much less likely to assign items to others outside the family. Figure 2.1A also shows a hypothetical distribution of items for normal children (Bene and Anthony, 1957) which suggests that the 'at-risk' group is much less like the normal pattern than the rest.

The second analysis compares the two groups of children in the way that each of the 40 items is given to family members. For 18 of the 40 items significant differences were found between the 'at-risk' and other children.

The most consistent trend across these findings was that the 'at-risk' children tend to express negative feelings about siblings but at the same time describe positive feelings coming from those same siblings. The others, in contrast, were less likely to express hostile feelings towards siblings and much more likely to describe positive feelings coming from mother. 'At-risk' children were also more likely to see negative incoming feelings from father than mother, although this was not a marked tendency for all relevant items.

Since consistent trends across some items can be found, the ability of these items to discriminate between the 'at-risk' and other children was tested by counting up

Distributions for:

A Hypothetical case (from Bene and Anthony, 1957)

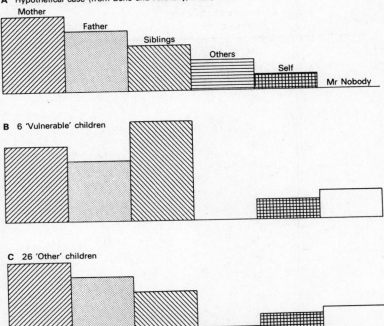

B 6 'Vulnerable' children

C 26 'Other' children

FIGURE 2.1   Allocation of items on the FRT to family and
non-family members

how many of these items were located by 'at-risk' and
other children in the expected place. By employing this
scoring framework, all children could be allocated a
'vulnerability' score, based on the types of locations of
items which appear to typify the 'vulnerable' group (i.e.
the 6 children scoring highest on visual contact). These
scores can range from −6 to +14. Table 2.12 shows the
distribution of scores for the 6 vulnerable and 26 other
children.

The distribution of scores in Table 2.12 shows that
these items, when scored in the way described, produce
a fairly accurate prediction of mother-contact style in
the strange situation, and therefore of response to the
hospital ward. Table 2.13 indicates that the degree of
accuracy is in the region of 93 per cent overall when
a cut-off of 8+ is employed. Efficiency of detecting true

TABLE 2.12   Distribution of 'vulnerability' scores on the basis of Bene-Anthony responses

Score	Vulnerability group*	Others
14	0	0
13	0	0
12	0	0
11	0	0
10	0	0
9	3	0
8	1	0
7	1	3
6	0	1
5	0	4
4	0	1
3	0	3
2	0	0
1	0	2
0	0	2
−1	0	3
−2	1	3
−3	0	2
−4	0	2
−5	0	0
−6	0	0

* Figures refer to the number of cases.

positives, however, is only 66 per cent, but efficiency at detecting true negatives is 100 per cent.

The generalised view of the 'vulnerable' child, therefore, is much more limited to family members, and contains highly ambivalent feelings about siblings. The not-at-risk child is much less ambivalent, and tends to include itself and non-family members in the family. The 'vulnerable' child's generalised view, therefore, is consistent with what had been observed by mother about

family interactions, namely that these children are much
more cohesively involved in family interaction, to the
exclusion of outsiders. The ambivalence of feelings about
other children in the family seems to be an integral part
of this greater involvement.

TABLE 2.13 Efficiency of 'vulnerability' scores

Using a cut-off of less than 8 as non-vulnerable:

	8+	7—
Vulnerables	4	2
Others	0	26

   Table 2.13 shows that some of the FRT items can be
used as an efficient and simple predictor of response to
strangeness and separation, but with considerable reserva-
tions at this stage. In the first place, it only predicts
mother-child contact in the strange situation and hence,
indirectly, the degree of overt upset during separation
in that situation. The value of the predictor is in
pointing to the kind of practical screening device that
might be used to detect children likely to be upset by
admission to hospital and to the form and aim of any such
device which might emerge from this study. The implication of this result seems to be that a measure of the
child's view of its own involvement in family dynamics
and the ambivalence of its feelings about siblings might
be a fruitful lead to the development of predictive
devices. The results reported here need to be cross-
validated on a second unselected sample in a hospital
setting before forming the basis of any practical screening procedure.

DISCUSSION

The weight of the evidence presented in this chapter
suggests that when the child is admitted to hospital,
depending on the patterns of the ward authority and the
limitations placed on the child through the characteristics
of the illness or condition, the child has to cope with
a certain degree of discontinuity of experience. By this
is meant that the child now has different expectations
placed on it, strange people to relate to, and familiar
people it is not able to relate to, or, even if the child
is able, the others, too, are affected by the discontinuity, and may respond to the child in unexpected ways.
The findings relating to family experiences suggest that

some children are much more disrupted by this discontinuity than others. The child who tends to remain in close contact with home, for example, becomes much more distressed. In contrast, the initiating child at home is not so distressed or withdrawn in hospital.

Children who are most distressed seem not only to come from high-proximity families but also to rely on direct visual contact with mother in certain situations and to be children who have mothers who are unquestioningly accepting of hospital authority. The high-initiating child, in contrast, is much more likely to use verbal modes of contact with mother in a strange situation and have a mother who only gives factual information in preparation, who visits less and who is generally not anxious about her child. Many of these relationships can be shown not only in the correlations reported here with hospital response but also appear when correlated with each other.

In the pilot study (Stacey et al., 1970) sociopsychiatric conclusions of the data collected at that time suggested that it might be worth while to think of the problems of children in hospital in terms of individual actors moving in and out of social systems which act upon them and which they in turn affect, rather than focus on the disruption of the bond with mother. A survey of the detailed and complicated data presented in this chapter suggests that this conclusion was well founded, and has pointed to some of the features of those systems which appear to be of most theoretical and practical relevance.

It is evident that this conclusion is partially founded upon assumptions that are contrary to those widely accepted and implicit in the writings and decision-taking of research workers and practitioners alike across the broad spectrum of child mental health. In particular, it seems contrary to the assumption that early experience is potent in the establishment of later patterns of behaviour. The Swansea team, however, is at this time not alone in questioning this widely accepted assumption and the reader is referred in particular to Clarke and Clarke (1976). This is not to say, of course, that it is of no importance as to what kinds of experiences the child has in infancy nor does the evidence presented in this chapter and in the remainder of this book imply any criticism of the self-evident humane effects that the writings of Bowlby and others had during the 1950s. As Clarke and Clarke argue, so forcefully, there is now beginning to be clear evidence that the whole of development is important, not merely development during the infant years.

In a general sense the speculative framework outlined
in the pilot study has received confirmation of its usefulness and relevance in this present study. Nevertheless,
the framework remains speculative to the extent that what
has been added to the original studies of children in
hospital has been the broadest outline of certain concepts
which, with much more research, might serve to provide
guidelines for concentrated research aimed at achieving
further progress in alleviating the problems of children
in hospital. The remaining chapters in this book explore
several other aspects of the model, and its implications.

CHAPTER THREE

The Validation of Meaning in Illness-Treatment Situations

Fred Clough

DISCREPANCY THEORY

The basic proposition, that an individual's interpretation of his situation is a primary determinant of his behaviour in that situation, has provided a major framework for the study of patienthood (Skipper and Leonard, 1965), but precise predictive models of this theoretical process have been little utilised in spite of their wide currency in the social sciences. In discussing the meaning of hospitalisation Coe (1970) predicts that:

> By and large, it would be expected that a patient's perception of his hospital experience would depend upon the degree of congruence between the model of care he expects to receive and what kind he is given in actual fact.... The greater the degree of congruence between the patient's expectations and his actual experience, the less traumatic the episode will be.

Coe's general proposition represents one of several conceptually similar approaches to social motivation, which may be loosely termed 'discrepancy theory'. The central problem in conceptualising this approach to meaning derives from a tendency to assume that situational meanings are either culturally determined and function as normative blueprints for action, or that they are primarily idio-syncratic to individual circumstances. Hence Herzlich (1973) complains that studies of illness behaviour have neglected the importance of the interaction between social meanings and individual interpretations of illness-treatment situations. This general problem is also subject to an extended discussion by Brittan (1973) who concludes: 'What really happens is that we work towards some practical compromise between what the imputed definition demands, and our actual perception of the situation. In so doing, we construct new meanings.' From the point of view of discrepancy theory, two conceptually distinct though functionally interacting sources of potential discontinuity appear to be involved in the construction of situational meaning. The first concerns the nature of social expectations established in one social system, as opposed to the normative standards of expectations defining some other systems; the two sets of standards may or may not match. The second source of discontinuity applies to the nature of the actual experiences, or 'perceptions' of those experiences, generated by encounters with different social systems; these encounters may also vary independently. Incongruity may therefore occur between expectancies, between more direct experiences, or between expectancies and experiences.

The discrepancy hypothesis is thus immensely complicated by this problem, and further complicated by the potential multi-dimensionality of the consequences of situational change and the problematic issue of their psychological organisation. What this analysis suggests, however, is that, as a first approximation, comparison standards may perhaps be conceived primarily as sociologically determined expectancies or *social definitions*; whilst *personal definitions* may refer to individual perceptions of events at a psychological level (see also Stebbins, 1971). The construction of meaning thus rests upon a compromise socio-psychological conception of incongruity.

A SOCIO-PSYCHOLOGICAL CONCEPTION

In the light of this brief discussion it is suggested that hospitalisation confronts both the child and adult patient with the problem of constructing a meaningful definition of his/her situation in the face of a potential social and conceptual discontinuity. It is not assumed that patients simply adopt normative cultural definitions regardless of their particular circumstances, nor is it assumed that individuals interpret the significance of their personally defined situations without reference to the commonly shared social standards by which they may be evaluated. Instead, a socio-psychological perspective is suggested in which the 'social validation of meaning' (Festinger, 1954) is dependent upon the attainment of an equilibrium, or compatibility, between personal and social definitions of the situation. It will be concerned with the nature of the match between 'what is' and 'what ought to be'. Moreover, it is assumed that the outcomes of this hypothetical comparison process will have significance for the individual's behaviour in a given situation. A more specific model of this conception may now be examined.

DEFINING THE SITUATION - FUNDAMENTAL MEANING

Medical sociologists have emphasised that illness-treatment
situations are socially defined and that the sick-patient
role essentially implies a social relationship defined by a
characteristic set of shared assumptions and mutual expectations. In a more phenomenological vein, McHugh (1968) refers
to the 'definition of the situation' as a sociological notion
analogous to the more general use of 'meaning'. Here there
is a concern with the organisation of meaning in social
interaction and with how orderly interaction is sustained
by shared assumptions concerning the means and ends of such
interaction.

In so far as McHugh is concerned with the process by which
meaning is organised (rather than with its content) this
conception offers a model of sufficient generality to be
potentially applicable to the analysis of illness behaviour
in varying situations, and even at different stages of
development. McHugh's analysis of the processes by which
social interaction is sustained, and how meaning and behaviour
are related, suggests in effect a form of discrepancy theory,
compatible with the socio-psychological conception introduced
above. He proposes that a social relationship is meaningful
to the extent that role partners continue to assume common
and intelligible means and ends. When these fundamental
assumptions are challenged for some reason, as when a
conversation proceeds at cross-purposes, the meaningfulness
of the social relationship will be threatened and interaction
may become disordered. An individual in these circumstances
may then re-examine his purposive assumptions and attempt to
re-establish a new basis for interaction. Where no satisfactory resolution of meaning is possible, the interaction
may be disrupted and may even be terminated, otherwise the
situation may degenerate into a state of meaninglessness,
anomie or alienation.

Whilst McHugh is primarily attempting to account for
the organisation of meaning and behaviour in an on-going
face-to-face interaction, such as a conversation, the
theoretical process which he suggests can perhaps be
generalised to social relationships in a much broader context.
Patienthood essentially implies a social relationship between
a sick person and his treatment agents. Whether it will be
a meaningful relationship will depend upon the extent to
which the participants can continue to share fundamental
assumptions concerning the social function of patienthood.
Hospitalisation is essentially an act of faith, resting upon
the fundamental social assumption that illness is undesirable
and medical treatment effective. Admission to hospital does
not validate these assumptions automatically: any commitment

is provisional upon a continued ability to define the
situation in terms of meaningful ends and means. On the
basis of unpredictable changes in the illness condition and
treatment procedures alone, these assumptions may be
challenged, and may have to be revised by the patient;
information extracted from direct communication, and personal
observations, will intrude in the continual process of
validation.

BEHAVIOURAL IMPLICATIONS OF VALIDATION

McHugh is quite clear about the psychological and behavioural
implications of how the individual is defining his situation
(1968, p. 135): 'Changes in definition will be accompanied
by changes in consequences.' If the fundamental assumptions
are confirmed, interaction is likely to be orderly and
meaningful; if they are refuted, the consequence will be
a disordered interaction and an experienced meaninglessness.
Moreover, he specifies that the validation of meaning is a
decision-making process involving a continual re-appraisal
of the means and ends of social interaction (1958, p. 50):
'The disorder of an interaction, then, hinges on a decision
by the actor that one or the other of these rules is
inoperative - that purpose is unintelligible or means
unavailable.' Since the validity of either ends or means, or
both, may be refuted, three kinds of disordered meanings
can be distinguished. Table 3.1 suggests how these
alternatives may be classified.

TABLE 3.1 Classification of means-ends relationships and
their validatory outcomes

	Means validated	Means invalidated
Ends validated	Meaningfulness	Powerlessness 'ends without means'
Ends invalidated	Purposelessness 'means without ends'	Meaninglessness 'without ends, without means'

The extent to which the validatory outcomes of Table 3.1
can be described in terms of qualitatively different
psychological states is briefly discussed by McHugh. An
alternative possibility is that these distinctions will be

quantitative, with the meaninglessness increasing with the
extent and degree of invalidation. From this point of view
meaninglessness will be more total and more likely to result
in decisive efforts to terminate the relationship, where
both means and ends are invalidated. But intermediate
positions, where both confirmation and refutation are involved
suggest states of indecision, where the social situation may
be sustained only at the cost of some ambivalence or conflict;
the behavioural concomitants of powerlessness and purposeless-
ness may therefore reflect emotional tension rather than an
unambiguous acceptance or rejection of interaction.

This line of analysis would bring McHugh's discrepancy
model into close agreement with similar conflict, incongruity
and dissonance models of motivation already well-established
in social psychology. Indeed, the similarity is quite
striking when we consider further McHugh's analysis of
emergence and relativity as dimensions of the validatory
process. Essentially, these processes express two major
ways in which personal definitions of current experiences
may be compared against various reference standards.

Emergence is a temporal dimension, and here the social
present may be compared against a current (or perceived)
meaning of the past or a current anticipation of the future.
For the hospital patient, therefore, the meaningfulness of
the present social situation can be validated in relation to
a standard of appropriateness derived from accustomed social
relationships in the past; it can also be validated against
the anticipation of prospects for the future, in relation to
expectancies of success or failure, expressed emotionally as
hopes and fears, as suggested by Feather (1963).

Relativity, on the other hand, is seen by McHugh as a
spatial dimension, involving the comparison of a present
event in its relationship to other events against the
immediate scene. Thus the patient may validate his conception
of himself against his perception of other patients, or he
may validate what he believes or has been told about his
illness and treatment against his own bodily feelings and
experiences. Personal definitions of the situation will thus
derive their relative meanings on the basis of a complex
decision-process involving the comparison and organisation of
many discrete events.

In other motivational discrepancy models, the problem of
how this match-mismatch comparison process should be
conceived has been a central theoretical issue. Most
cognitive-motivational models assume that current events are
either compared amongst themselves or against some other
standard, and that the perception of a discrepancy will have
motivational consequences for the organism (Harvey, 1963).
The nature of the mismatch discrepancy has been variously

described in relationship terms, as cognitive inconsistency, incongruity, uncertainty, imbalance, conflict or dissonance (Berlyne, 1965). In behavioural terms it has been assumed to have outcomes in expressions of emotionality, or in instrumental attempts to reduce the discrepancy in some way, by exploration, information-seeking, or escape from the situation.

PREDICTION AND EVALUATION

Underlying these alternative formulations are two distinct dimensions of psychological discrepancy which should not be confused. In the first place 'a discrepancy' suggests a perceived difference between a situation as encountered and as expected; here we may refer to the experiences of incongruity, surprise or uncertainty, that is, to the predictability of social expectations. In the second place, 'a discrepancy' will usually indicate additionally a change in how a current situation is appraised against some evaluative reference standard, whether it involves a change for the better or for the worse, rather than merely a change *per se*. Here we are concerned with the directional implications of social interaction, for the experience of value-loss or value-gain, and for approach, avoidance, or conflictual tendencies, as alternative behavioural consequencies.

Many studies of patienthood, however, have emphasised the predictability function of informational communications, without regard to any implied directionality. For example, it is often argued that the patient should 'know the truth' about his illness and treatment predicament, and that otherwise psychological uncertainty will be a maladaptive outcome. In the same way, the problem of meaning for the very young child is generally considered to be one of coping with the unfamiliarity and unpredictability of the hospital setting. Whilst the ability to organise on-going experiences, locate goals and predict outcomes may be a necessary condition for effective adaptation, it cannot be a sufficient condition without regard to the directional implications of a cognitive appraisal. The plea, 'Where am I, where am I going, what are they doing to me?', is not only a cry for information but is a cry for a reassurance that the means and ends of interaction will have positive rather than negative consequences.

DEFINING THE STANDARD: DISSONANCE MODELS

The problem of the alternative predictability and
directionality dimensions of match-mismatch relationships
is closely associated with the problem of how we might
define the nature of the 'standard' against which on-going
experiences are to be compared, and from which they derive
their meaning. McHugh's discussion of emergence, in which
standards are vested in past experience or future anticipation,
and of relativity, in which current events are compared
amongst themselves, is essentially a proposal for a variety
of relevant standards. It may now be argued that there are
some standards relevant to the predictability of events, and
others primarily relevant to their directionality or evaluation; in a more complex analysis, both dimensions may be
implicated in the same reference standard.

In a related context, Festinger (1957) has proposed a
discrepancy hypothesis which gives explicit recognition to
the problem of different reference standards. The
discrepancy relationship with which Festinger is concerned
is that of cognitive dissonance. Dissonant relations may
occur not only between two cognitions but also between a
cognition and a behavioural act; in the latter case the
person may now, for example, perceive that he has behaved
inappropriately, in the light of a re-definition of the
consequences of that action, so that he may regret it:
'The two elements are in a dissonant relation if, considering
these two alone, the obverse of one element would follow
from the other.' Dissonant relations therefore occur where
there are non-fitting or non-matching elements which do not
'make sense' together.

Festinger suggests a number of ways in which dissonance
could arise. It could arise from a logical inconsistency,
as when a person maintains logically contradictory beliefs.
It could arise because of the existence of cultural standards
prescribing what ought to be believed, valued or enacted;
the dissonance exists simply because the culture defines
what is consonant and what is not, with reference to widely
shared value assumptions. Finally, dissonance may arise
from standards established by past expectancies; the person
knows from experience what to expect (i.e. what follows what,
in the predictability sense) and if this empirical expectancy
is disconfirmed he experiences cognitive dissonance. Hence
there is some attempt to distinguish between logical,
evaluative (directional) and empirical (predictability)
bases for dissonant relations, each associated with different
reference standards.

DISSONANCE AND HOSPITAL TREATMENT

Going to hospital is an experience which is potentially
liable to arouse cognitive dissonance (Festinger) or threaten
meaningfulness (McHugh). Taken together, both conceptions
suggest that the hospital experience may be validated (or
invalidated) against a variety of reference standards. In
the first place, hospitalisation may be socially defined in
terms of widely shared assumptions of appropriate and valued
means and ends of interaction. These social definitions
or standards always involve consonant cognitions according
to a social logic or rule system for what 'makes sense' in
illness-treatment situations. For example, being a hospital
patient implies that one is ill (the removal of illness is
the goal) and that treatment will be to some extent effective
as a means. This assumption may be challenged, however, by
personal definitions implying alternative and incompatible
means-ends relationships, as discussed by McHugh.

Rationality, in the conventional logical sense, can
provide yet another rule system for validating personal
definitions. If a patient believes that medical treatment
will be effective, yet also believes that the illness
condition is incurable, these cognitions are logically
contradictory. Other problems of logical dissonance may
arise because an individual's own system of implication is
not strictly valid in the logical sense. A child, for
example, may believe that because a treatment procedure is
painful or stressful, then it is therefore disfunctional;
on the other hand, the child may believe that a treatment
is functional because it is not stressful, or even that it is
functional because it is stressful. Adults are not immune
to such logical fallacies: when parents were asked how
they would choose between long and stressful hospital
treatment as opposed to a short, stressful treatment for
their child, given the same illness condition (scoliosis),
some parents admitted that they would choose the long-stay
treatment since it must be the more effective (Clough, 1975).
In fact, unknown to the parents, such alternatives existed
but there was no evidence for a clinical consensus concerning
their respective merits.

A final reference standard is empirical rather than
logical. Present situations may be validated on no other
basis than that they conform to the familiar pattern of
prior experiences. The appeal to the familiar may have
neither a rational necessity nor a social necessity, but
it may reflect a consistent rule system nevertheless. Here
the reference standard is to be found not in how the current
situation is socially defined but in how a prior reference
situation is socially defined. A young child, for example,

may find the hospital experience incompatible with his/her prior social experiences in the family. The match between 'what is' and 'what ought to be' is now based upon social assumptions appropriate to past situations, rather than those appropriate to present means and future goals. It is true that both sets of expectations will be derived from prior experiences, but the essential distinction here is between a comparison which is either retrospectively or prospectively orientated. On the one hand an individual may invest value priorities in the past, whilst on the other he/she may be able to forgo past satisfactions and give priority to future goals. It is in this sense, perhaps, that McHugh finds it necessary to give a greater emphasis to what he calls 'definitional time' as opposed to chronological time; the former takes into account this dual time perspective.

In addition to the conceptual similarities between how McHugh, Festinger and other discrepancy theorists define the nature of potential reference standards, there is considerable agreement concerning the implications of such discrepancies for behaviour. McHugh refers rather generally to 'disordered interaction' as a consequence of meaninglessness. Festinger and other cognitive consistency theorists typically suggest that dissonance will be associated with a state of uncomfortable psychological tension and that a person will be motivated to reduce dissonance and restore consistency. This may be achieved by modifying discrepant beliefs in order to justify one's behaviour, or by changing one's behaviour to match one's beliefs, as in attempting to escape from the dissonance-producing situation altogether.

In this context there are certain important characteristics of hospitalisation that are likely to increase the potential for dissonance arousal and yet decrease the potential for its reduction. In the first place hospitalisation is frequently an involuntary event for the individual, as well as a sudden and unfamiliar event, so that there is often the likelihood that admission involves a public enactment without a private commitment. In the second place, hospitalisation is usually a social act that the patient cannot readily reverse. The patient may thus be committed to a course of action which is dissonant with his/her personal definition of the situation (e.g. he/she may regret it), but he/she may be unable to reduce an uncomfortable state of dissonance by reversing this action, either because such a decision is not possible or because it would involve other serious consequences. Festinger has investigated experimentally the situation of 'forced compliance' or 'insufficient justification' from a dissonance point of view, with results suggesting that the individual may sometimes reduce dissonance 'by coming to value the things

for which he has suffered'. Where dissonance cannot be
resolved in such ways, however, the situation can become
intolerable and anxiety-provoking, and disorders of meaning
and social interaction may be inevitable, as McHugh suggests.

TWO PROPOSITIONS

Festinger's discussion of the sources of cognitive
dissonance, and McHugh's analysis of emergence and relativity
in the validation of meanings, are complementary. Both are
concerned with how the individuals are continually re-defining
their personal situation and comparing current experiences
against a variety of reference standards. The notion of the
match-mismatch process in discrepancy theory is thus
complicated by the variety of potential standards and their
multi-dimensionality. Nevertheless it has perhaps usefully
widened the scope of the basic proposition, that individuals
validate their personal definitions of a situation with
reference to some social standard or rule system. That
several validatory processes are implicated is only to be
expected.
    A second basic proposition, that the validation or non-
validation of meaning has important consequences for
behaviour, is also considered by these two theorists. A
failure to validate appropriate and valued means and ends
of interaction is likely to be associated with aversive
psychological states and emotionally negative behaviours
involving anxiety or hostility. It was argued previously
that in the hospital context these potentially maladaptive
reactions might depend upon either a degree of conflict
(anxiety) or unambiguous rejection (hostility), which are
likely to be involved where a current situation is personally
defined as incompatible with a variety of reference standards.
Hence partial invalidations of assumptions (e.g. 'means
without ends', or 'ends without means') suggest conflicts
of meanings; whilst more total invalidations, in which both
ends and means are incompatible with social assumptions,
suggest meaninglessness and an unambiguous rejection of
the social relationship. These differential behavioural
outcomes are not made explicit by McHugh but are further
possible predictions derived from a psychological analysis
of conflict and frustration (Barker et al., 1953).

MEANING AND BEHAVIOUR - A STUDY OF OLDER CHILDREN IN HOSPITAL

The study of the meaning of hospitalisation for older child
patients, and its relationship to behaviour, is not only

valid in its own right but also has its rationale within a
wider developmental perspective. Moreover, the investigation
of meaning within the framework of discrepancy theory may be
facilitated by the employment of measurement techniques well
established in research with adults but relatively un-
developed for use with young children. Hopefully, however,
such techniques could be subsequently modified and extended
systematically downwards through the age range.

I adopted this strategy in a study of 104 female
orthopaedic inpatients (aged from 9 to 16 years) distributed
through three children's wards in three different hospitals
(Clough, 1975). Biographical variables, diagnosis, immediate
treatment conditions and current length of stay varied
widely but were 'measured' for each individual. The child's
perception of aspects of her illness, treatment, home, and
ward environment (her 'psychological space') was assessed
in situ using the semantic differential technique (Osgood
et al., 1957). Each child judged each of 16 important
concepts relating to hospital and self against a standard
set of 24 bipolar adjective-rating scales. At the time
of assessment, staff ratings of the child's recent and
characteristic behaviour in the ward were also obtained.

The primary objective of the research was to explore the
nature of the relationship between (a) a structure of
background and situational events, (b) a structure of
personal meanings and (c) a structure of observed behaviours
in the ward. It was guided first by the general hypothesis
that at this age level the cultural meaning of hospitalisation
for the group would reflect an organised adult-like social
definition, as described by medical sociologists. Further,
it was hypothesised that individual variations in personal
definitions of the conceptual environment would predict
patient behaviours on the basis of a discrepancy theory;
that is, disorders of behaviour would be associated with
disorders of meaning, in which the patient defined her
personal situation as in conflict with, or incompatible
with, the assumptions of a meaningful and purposeful social
relationship.

DIMENSIONS OF MEANING

The technical aspects of this study are given in Clough (1975)
and cannot be described here in detail. Factor analysis
was employed to reduce the dimensionality of each of the
three large data sets to its basic independent components.
A first task was to establish the major dimensions of
meaning contained in the 24 specific rating judgments of
the semantic differential scales. A first rotated Varimax

factor analysis revealed that, regardless of specific
concepts, the children had in effect structured their
situation in terms of three independent dimensions of
meaning:
  (i) (E) High v. Low Functional Evaluation (good/bad,
        helpful/harmful, safe/unsafe, etc.)
 (ii) (P) High v. Low Predictability/Familiarity (well-known/
        strange, certain/uncertain, understandable/puzzling,
        etc.)
(iii) (S) High v. Low Stress/Restriction (strict/easygoing,
        tight/loose, painful/not painful, etc.)

THE CULTURAL MEANING OF HOSPITALISATION

The construct validity of these provisional interpretations
depends further upon whether the three response dimensions
can differentiate the concept space in a meaningful way.
A statistical cluster analysis revealed that this was so.
The 16 concepts reduced to four major clusters or concept
areas, whose meanings were defined by different combinations
of the three response dimensions (E,P,S). These independent
areas of the conceptual space could confidently be identified
as Home Life, Ward Life, Medical Treatment and Illness.
    Figure 3.1 illustrates the nature of these clusters as
they appear graphically, for example in the the two-
dimensional space formed by the response dimensions of
Functional Evaluation (E) and Stress/Restriction (S). The
cultural meaning of the four primary concept areas can be
summarised by the mean judgment for the total sample, as
further shown in Figure 3.2.
    The semantic differential analysis reveals a multi-
dimensional system with a meaningful differentiation of
the patients' conceptual environment. The cultural
meaning of the four primary 'concerns' of patients may
therefore be defined in the following way:
 Home Life: Functional (E+), Not Stressful(S—),
            Predictable (P+)
 Ward Life: Disfunctional (E—), Not Stressful (S—),
            Unpredictable (P—)
 Medical Treatment: Functional (E+), Stressful (S+),
                    Unpredictable (P—)
 Illness: Disfunctional (E—), Stressful (S+),
          Predictable (P+)
    It is of some interest to note that when analysis was
carried out separately for each of the three hospital
samples involved, the structures of semantic differential
dimensions and of concept space were essentially equivalent.
Figure 3.2 therefore describes highly generalised meanings

representative of the orthopaedic patient culture at this age range. This does not preclude, of course, significant individual variations amongst patients, nor between more specific illness-treatment situations.

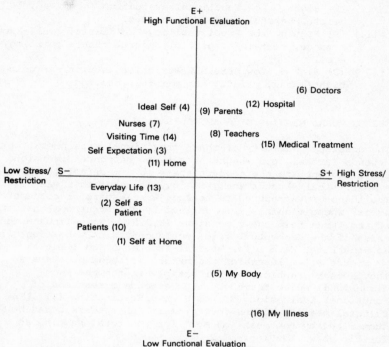

Standardised mean factor scores for total patient sample (N = 104)

FIGURE 3.1   Semantic differential concept space: group concept means for Evaluation by Stress (Varimax factors)

(a) Functional Evaluation by Stress

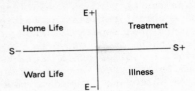

(b) Functional Evaluation by Predictability

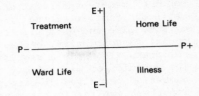

(c) Predictability by Stress

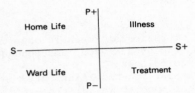

FIGURE 3.2 The cultural meaning of primary concept areas (based on total sample mean scores)

PERCEIVED DISCREPANCIES

The usefulness of these structures of meaning is hardly in doubt. In the first place the three response dimensions – Evaluation, Predictability and Stress reflect conceptually distinct aspects of psychological influence central to the patient experience, yet usually inextricably confounded and devoid of empirical referents in the global hospital situation. In the second place in defining the cultural meanings of concepts, the various combinations of dimensional values have not only an obvious face validity but a considerable power to demonstrate important theoretical contrasts suggested by discrepancy theory. Home Life, which is identified with the Ideal Self, suggests a reference standard with which the other three concept areas are directly contrasted (along the diagonals of Figure 3.2). Hence, in contrast with Home Life, Illness is typically disfunctional and stressful, Ward Life disfunctional and unpredictable, and Medical Treatment stressful and unpredictable.

There is evidence, however, that these children (as a whole) are able to construct realistic ambivalent conceptions of Medical Treatment (as functional yet stressful and un-predictable), suggesting a mature mode of conceptualisation unlikely to be available to younger patients. This hypothesis leads in the direction of a Piagetian analysis of concept development, and suggests also that McHugh's model of means-ends relationships can be perhaps operationally defined.   Similarly, the direct contrast between the meanings of Home Life and Ward Life suggests that separation and social discontinuity, emphasised in the study of young children, also have a significance for older child patients. The dynamics of meaning may thus be analysed in terms of a number of perceived discrepancies which are assumed to have important implications for the prediction of patient behaviour.

THE DIMENSIONS OF OBSERVED BEHAVIOUR

In order to test this general hypothesis, staff ratings (nurses and teachers combined) of patients' recently observed behaviour in the ward were also factor analysed, and reduced to four independent dimensions as follows:
  (i) Non-Compliance v. Compliance: Non-Compliant children were more disobedient, unco-operative, disrespectful, quarrelsome and bad tempered.
 (ii) High v. Low Emotional Anxiety: Anxious children were reported as more easily upset, miserable, tense and withdrawn.
(iii) Expressive v. Inhibited: Expressive children asked questions concerning their illness, treatment and hospital life. They expressed their feelings, showed curiosity, were sociable, often to the extent of showing-off.
 (iv) High v. Low Ego Strength: Children scoring high were reported as 'acting superior', displaying leadership, self-confidence, stability, independence and alertness.
   It should be noted that the dimensions of non-compliance and anxiety behaviour, as defined here, follow closely a well-established distinction in the clinical literature between 'conduct problems' and 'personality problems' (Quay and Quay, 1965). Expressiveness corresponds to the well-known Extraversion/Introversion factor of Eysenck (1952), which has been frequently replicated. The significance of this classification is further supported by an almost identical factor-structure of teachers' ratings of children's classroom behaviour, reported by Herbert (1974). There can therefore be some confidence in the validity of the four-dimensional structure adopted here.

DIMENSIONS OF LIFE-HISTORY AND SITUATIONAL INFLUENCES

A detailed schedule of information concerning each patient's

family background, age, level of educational attainment,
illness and hospitalisation history, current length of stay
and current treatment programme was compiled from interview
data, hospital records and direct observation in the ward.
These data were also subject to factor analysis in order to
establish the major independent sources of variance. The
assumption here is that, underlying many specific social and
situational characteristics, will be a small number of basic
factors representative of important sources of influence on
patient perceptions and behaviour. The outcome of these
analyses is briefly summarised by the variables entered into
the left-hand side of Figure 3.3, where each box represents
independent factors formed by weighted combinations of
specific measurements reflected in the overall factor-
scores. More precise detail is found in Clough (1975). Any
subsequent reference to background and situational 'influence'
will be a reference to these factor-dimensions.

THE RELATIONSHIP BETWEEN STRUCTURES: METHODS OF ANALYSIS

The major objective is to explore the nature of the general
relationships between three structures of independent
dimensions - between environmental influence, semantic-
differential 'meanings', and observed behaviour.   In practice
it was necessary to approach this complex multi-variate
problem through the analysis of pairs of structures rather
than all three simultaneously. The methods of factor
analysis, multiple regression, path analysis and canonical
correlation (Cooley and Lohnes, 1971) were used to this
purpose. More specific lines of relationship between single
variables were also analysed using correlational procedures,
and sub-group differences and interactions were selectively
explored using t-test statistics. Many of these procedures
are alternatives and only a brief selection will be
considered in order to convey the emergent common findings.

CORRELATES OF PATIENT BEHAVIOUR

The test of the general hypothesis - that patients'
perceptions of their situation are related to their observed
behaviours in the ward - is a rigorous one, in so far as
the patients' semantic-differential responses and the staff
behaviour-rating measures were obtained from independent
sources. The two sets of scores were intercorrelated and
the main results can be briefly reported by reference to
statistically significant levels for r (product correlation
coefficient) and R (multiple correlation coefficient), as

appropriate.   Background and situational factors also enter
into this analysis.

Observed Compliant behaviour correlated with two
major independent sources.   First, the perception of Illness
as predictably disfunctional (E—P+), a measure of the
tendency 'to define oneself as ill', related to Compliance
(R=0.30, p < 0.01).   Second, children of higher educational
status (with other social-class indicators such as occupational status and family size controlled) were also independently rated more Compliant by ward staff (r=0.27,
p < 0.01).

Observed Anxiety behaviour was also found to have two
major subjective correlates, suggesting an important
distinction between Social and Treatment Anxiety: where
Ward Life (low evaluation) was unfavourably contrasted with
Home Life (high), Anxiety behaviour was more evident
(R=0.32, p < 0.01).   Where Medical Treatment was perceived
as stressful and disfunctional, Anxiety behaviour was again
correlated (R=0.32, p < 0.01);   in addition, perceptions
of Treatment as disfunctional were made more frequently by
children rated low in Ego Strength (or Low Morale).
Reported Anxiety behaviour was also independently correlated
with physical stress factors in the environment, such as
the rated degree of restrictive plaster treatment (r=0.32,
p < 0.01).

Expressive or Socially Extraverted behaviours tended to
increase in the sample generally as current length of
hospital stay increased (r=0.19, p=0.05);   similarly, Peer
Popularity, assessed from patients' friendship choices,
also increased significantly as a function of both length
of stay and age.   Taken together, these findings suggest
that sociability was related to familiarisation with the
group setting - as a function of time in the ward - and that
age facilitated this process so far as peer adjustment was
concerned;   sociability, on the present criteria, appears
to be an independent dimension of adjustment unrelated to
illness-treatment perceptions and their emotional
concomitants.

THE PATH ANALYSIS

Figure 3.3 is a path diagram (Mapes and Allen, 1973)
showing all the significant linear relationships linking
four major sets of time-sequenced variables.   All the shown
paths (arrows) are marked with standardised regression
coefficients, indicating independent components of
'determination' at a statistically significant level
(p < 0.05).   The coefficients were established by the method

of repeated regression analysis, whereby each variable was
in turn regressed on to all other variables preceding it in
the assumed time sequence. On the basis of this analysis,
the arrows suggest direct causal linkage between variables.
Of primary theoretical interest is the relative failure of
the assessments of background influences (such as prior
illness, hospitalisation and family status) to predict
patient behaviour directly. It is the semantic-differential
perceptions (personal definitions), and immediate treatment
variables, which show significant relationships of a *direct*
kind. However, in so far as some background characteristics
do relate significantly to patient perceptions, which in
turn predict behaviour, a mediational model is suggested:
prior experiences will have a modifying effect on how the
patient will define her situation, and thus influence
behaviour *indirectly*.

The most important 'background characteristic' is undoubtedly the child's level of educational attainment (with
age controlled). It is of some interest that low educational
level is itself significantly associated with low family
social status and with high prior hospitalisation (frequency
and duration), and these are assumed to be causal factors.
There is thus evidence that repeated or prolonged hospitalisa-
sation can have a disruptive effect on educational progress
but that congenital orthopaedic handicap (without hospitalisation) need not have such consequences. When all other background variables are controlled educational level also shows
significant correlation with treatment perceptions. In
brief, children of high educational level tend to define
medical treatment as functional yet stressful, whilst those
of lower educational level tend to define treatment as less
stressful but disfunctional; if it can be assumed that
educational level offers a rough indicator of differential
cognitive maturity within this age group, then greater
cognitive maturity is associated with a more adult-like
ambivalent definition of medical treatment, a finding
predictable on the basis of cognitive developmental theory,
and supported by the results of a study by Campell (1975).

The correlational findings therefore suggest that the
greater compliance observed amongst children of higher
educational level in the present sample is mediated by a
greater stress-tolerance, which derives from the priority
they tend to give to long-term functional outcomes of
medical treatment, in spite of its shorter-term stressful
consequences. Their definition of the treatment situation
thus reveals a blend of faith and realism, a stance which
perhaps matches an 'ambivalent standard' of the medical
culture, expressed by the dictum that 'Sometimes it is
necessary to be cruel to be kind.'

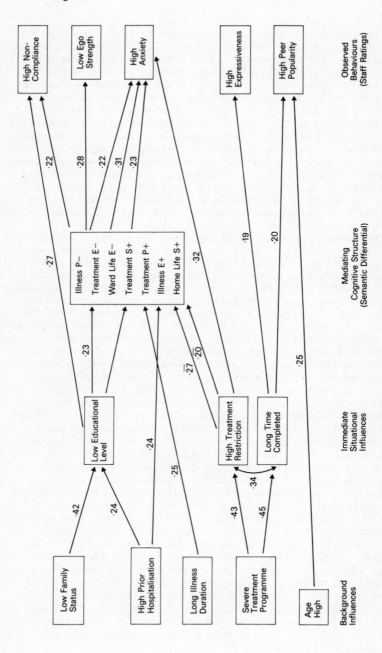

FIGURE 3.3 Path analysis assuming a causal interpretation of patient behaviour

INTERPRETATION OF DISFUNCTIONAL PERCEPTIONS OF ILLNESS

It can also be shown from Figure 3.3 that low prior
hospitalisation and high current treatment restriction
correlate significantly with a tendency to perceive illness
as more disfunctional. A first interpretation of this
relationship suggests that the three variables are linked
to a particular diagnostic group, such as idiopathic
scoliosis, a deforming orthopaedic condition of rapid late
onset requiring a relatively severe and prolonged plaster
restriction. This may be so but nevertheless it is the
treatment characteristics that are important, rather than,
for example, illness duration.

A discontinuity interpretation is also plausible. The
more severe the treatment, the greater the likelihood that
hospitalisation will be discontinuous with the patient's
prior experience, especially if the patient has never been
in hospital before. In combination, the absence of prior
hospitalisation and the presence of high current restriction
actually indicate a situation where the least experienced
patients are encountering the most severe treatment conditions;
discontinuity of treatment career (see Pill, ch.6) may
arouse a greater sensitivity towards illness as a threat -
that is, relative to the norm of 'health' which governs the
outside world, rather than relative to the norm of 'illness'
which governs the culture of the hospital. A further
relevant explanation concerns the nature of the cues which
are made available to patients on the basis of changes in
their treatment programme. To be put to bed is to be defined
as ill, to be re-mobilised is to be defined as at least
partly recovered. These cues may not in fact correlate with
clinical judgment but they may be all that patients have
if they are to define their current condition. The problem
of how the sick person comes to re-define his/her condition
through successive stages of the sick-patient role has of
course preoccupied students of illness behaviour (Suchman,
1965a, 1965b; Robinson, 1971). Changes in treatment
procedures are likely to be strongly implicated in this
definitional process.

It can be argued that a linear correlational analysis
is not the most appropriate from the point of view of a
mediational model, nor from the point of view of a discrepancy
theory. Whilst it provides a useful general picture of
additive influences on behaviour, it leaves out of account
the potentially numerous complex interactions between perceptions, which are essential for the analysis of conceptual
conflict and dissonance. An attempt was therefore made to
analyse the relationship between particular combinations of
semantic-differential variables and behaviour ratings,
guided by theoretical considerations.

PREDICTING TREATMENT MOTIVATION

On the basis of McHugh's theory (see Table 3.1) the patient's definition of means-ends relationships will be reflected primarily in how she combines her conceptions of Illness and Medical Treatment. It is proposed that 'being a patient' assumes a purposeful 'goal' and appropriate 'means' to the extent that when the patient defines herself as ill she is also able to evaluate her medical treatment favourably, either in functional or in emotional terms. Given this personal definition, her treatment motivation should be positive, whilst the contrasting reverse definition suggests a negative treatment motivation (see Figure 3.4).

A second combination of means-ends relationships will reflect conceptual conflict, where the situation is defined as 'ends without means' or 'means without ends'. The former, where the patient defines herself as ill and yet devalues her treatment, suggests a motivational conflict, in which the tendencies to accept and simultaneously reject treatment are incompatible. On the other hand, the incongruous perception, 'means without ends', whilst not suggestive of a positive motivational state, hardly suggests a negative motivation or an emotional conflict; instead, it indicates a state of low or neutral motivation in which the patient defines herself as 'not ill' and her treatment as functional and non-stressful; it is therefore a definition of perceived recovery, satisfaction, or 'motivational relief' (Feather, 1963).

TESTING THE DISCREPANCY MODEL: SUB-GROUP COMPARISONS

Whilst McHugh associates incompatible and incongruous means-ends relationships (disorders of meaning) with 'disorders of behaviour' in a general sense, the above analysis suggests two major disorders of meaning with potentially different behavioural outcomes. There are two bases for comparing contrasting groups: positive treatment motivation versus negative treatment motivation, and high conflict versus low conflict; Figure 3.4 shows the structure of these suggested means-ends relationships. It should be noted that the analysis is for the moment confined to inter-actions between Illness and Treatment perceptions on the dimensions of Functional Evaluation and Stress; other concepts and other dimensions could be introduced, though the prediction of their theoretical and behavioural significance is more problematic.

The factor analysis of staff ratings of patient behaviour had revealed two relevant dimensions of behavioural

disturbance in the wards (Non-Compliance and Anxiety). It
was therefore possible not only to predict that the disorders
of meaning suggested by (a) and (c) of Figure 3.4 would be
related to reported disturbances of behaviour, but also to
predict the alternative behaviours.

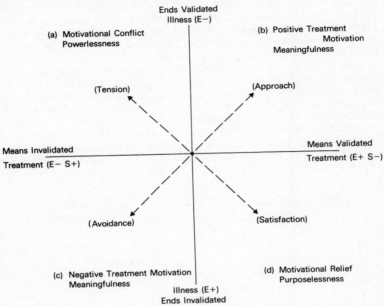

FIGURE 3.4 Means-ends relationships described by dimensions
of motivation and conflict

   Patients were divided into four sub-groups on the basis
of their patterns of illness-treatment evaluations, as shown
in Figure 3.4, and predictions of sub-group difference in
behaviour were made as follows:
   (i) Group (a) (High Motivational Conflict) should be rated
        higher in Anxiety behaviour than sub-group (d).
  (ii) Group (c) (Negative Treatment Motivation) should be
        rated in Non-Compliant, unco-operative and hostile
        behaviour than sub-group (b).
 (iii) Groups (a) and (c) should differ significantly on
        both the Anxiety and Non-Compliant behaviour
        dimensions.
   These sub-group comparisons were statistically analysed
for all cross-classifications of illness-treatment conceptions
on the three semantic-differential dimensions (EPS), using
one-tailed t-tests. Two points should be noted. First, all

cross-classifications involved statistically independent
(EPS) measures, and similarly the two behaviour ratings were
statistically independent of each other. Second, the prior
linear correlational analyses had discovered significant
correlations between illness perceptions and behaviour only
for the single relationship between Illness P+ and Compliance
(Figure 3.3). However, genuine interaction effects are now
predicted, on the basis that the meanings of Illness and
Medical Treatment are best defined in terms of a joint
interactive means-ends relationship.

The results of the sub-group comparisons strongly
confirmed all the predictions for cross-classifications
involving the functional dimension of Illness perceptions
(Illness E+,E—) when combined with judgment of Treatment
Evaluation and Stress (Treatment E, S). Figure 3.5 shows
the actual outcomes for behaviour in two primary structures
of means-ends relationships; in each case all predictions
were confirmed at a level of statistical significance of at
least p=0.05.

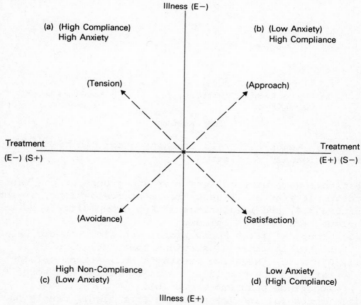

N.B. These observed behavioural outcomes should be compared
     with the theoretical structures shown in Figure 3.4.

FIGURE 3.5 Patterns of observed behaviour for major
semantic-differential sub-groups

These findings generally suggest that the children's definitions of their illness and treatment situations should not be considered in isolation but in terms of a 'psycho-social logic' of means-ends relationships, along the lines proposed by McHugh.

A MEDIATIONAL MODEL OF MEANING

The complexity of the mediational model suggested by the earlier correlational analysis is now apparent. There is an important sense in which a knowledge of any particular concept meaning does not allow the prediction of patient behaviour, but we need to know the rule system by which disparate elements of meaning are organised. In the linear path analysis (Figure 3.3), for example, no significant relationships were revealed between evaluative definitions of Illness and patient behaviour; but in interaction with Treatment perceptions, Illness emerges as a critical concept in the present analysis by virtue of its decisive contribution to a means-ends relationship. Meaning is thus not so much a reflection of events and influences but the outcome of a radical transformation and reorganisation, a construction of order according to some principle. It is in this sense that the term 'psycho-social logic' has been employed to the process of validating meaning.

   There is consistent and striking evidence that disorders of behaviour are related to disorders of meaning, described in terms of conceptual conflict, incongruity and dissonance, whilst emotional stability and compliance are related to cognitive consistency and meaningfulness. *In no case was a significant opposing relationship found.* Moreover, the child's definition of her hospital situation was a better predictor of her observed behaviour than the remaining (apparently quite powerful) background and situational factors combined (see Figure 3.3).

   Finally, it must be admitted that these findings can be interpreted variously as the effects of conceptions upon behaviour, of behaviour upon conceptions, or as a mutually interactive relationship. The assumption that meaning mediates behaviour can itself be challenged. However, it has provided a useful hypothesis for the present study, and one which may be briefly considered again from a developmental perspective.

DEVELOPMENTAL ASPECTS OF INTERPRETIVE PROCESSES

An attempt has been made to consider in theoretical and

empirical terms McHugh's proposition that disorders of
meaning and of behaviour tend to go together. Piaget (1967)
similarly asserts that 'the way the child is able to think
about people and events underlies the way he acts and feels
towards them'. It will not be possible to consider in
detail the full implications of a discrepancy theory of
meaning from a developmental perspective, though many studies
of children in hospital are relevant to this theme (Clough,
1973). The present discussion must be limited to certain
general developmental issues raised by the present emphasis
on the potential discontinuities of meaning inherent in
hospitalisation.

A central problem in the earlier analysis concerned how
we should conceptualise and locate the nature of an internal
standard of reference upon which to base the 'discrepancy
hypothesis'. A number of alternative proposals was
considered equally valid, though a distinction was made
between social standards located retrospectively in prior
social situations and those located prospectively in
anticipated outcomes. The constructs of social definition
and social expectation appear to refer to both time perspectives, and McHugh and Festinger have given recognition to
these possibilities.

A possible interpretation of developmental studies
suggests that a change in social standards for the validation
of meaningful interaction is likely to be dependent upon
general changes in cognitive social development. It is
suggested that the young child can derive a meaningful
present from activities which preserve the assumptions of
the past; the older child and adult additionally can derive
a meaningful present from the valued possibilities of the
future. This change in time perspective certainly reflects
a widely accepted generalisation about the normative course
of cognitive growth: 'The adolescent differs from the child
above all in that he thinks beyond the present' (Inhelder
and Piaget, 1958, p. 338). Clearly, both kinds of social
expectations can only become established as a result of
prior socialisation, but it is the time perspective which
distinguishes the change in the location of social reference
standards in this sense.

There is, therefore, a possible developmental resolution
to the problem of where to locate the notion of a primary
reference standard in discrepancy theory. The suggested
developmental progression is one in which the child's
interactions become less involved with the immediately
perceptible features of his/her environment and more with
a conceptual environment of beliefs and values. Kelvin
(1969) similarly characterises developmental changes in the
socialisation process: 'The child learns how to act before

he can understand the values which justify adult demands;
the more mature individual frequently starts with a set of
values which then determines how he acts.'

In the case of separation distress in infancy cognitive
processes become increasingly more significant in the
validation of meaning. When the child becomes developmentally
mature enough to recognise the separation from mother as a
discrepant event, the child's social standards for meaningful
interaction may be partly or completely refuted. This
discrepancy involves a standard vested in past familiar
experiences.

For the young child, with his standards rooted in the
past, the social discontinuities encountered in the moves
into and out of hospital suggest further challenges for the
child's ability to validate his experiences. These problems
extend beyond those of separation in infancy to include a
wider problem where expectations shaped in one social system
are or are not fulfilled when he moves into another system.
Hospitalisation is but one of a number of potential interruptions to the normal course of socialisation in childhood
(Moore, 1969), and social discontinuity essentially suggests
such interruption. Kelvin (1969) conceived the process of
socialisation as one which is functional for the individual
in so far as it facilitates his intrinsic information-
processing activities: 'To achieve this the environment
must be fairly stable, consistent or orderly; and to
manipulate or control it one must be able to make predictions;
if the situation is continually changing one cannot learn
from it nor use experience as a guide to the future.'

DISCONTINUITY IN HOSPITAL

A major theme of social discontinuity, therefore, might
be that going into hospital greatly increases the probability
that the social environment will become unpredictable for
the child. But a hospital can be unpredictable for children
in different ways, at different stages of cognitive
development and in relation to differing prior social
experiences. Not only will young children be cut off from
what is most familiar to them, but they will be exposed to
new and strange experiences. Moreover, hospital is a place
where the opportunities for exploration and information-
search are likely to be considerably reduced. Confinement
to bed tends to reduce social interactions which are a major
source of information, and much of what is important goes
on 'back-stage' anyway. There are also considerable
limitations to the hospital ward as a socialisation setting,
since the role of the patient is not clearly specified. The

patient is not usually instructed in what he/she should or
should not do, nor in what to expect from others (see Pill,
ch. 6).   It is important to remember also that an efficiently
structured routine in a hospital ward does not necessarily
imply a highly predictable environment - since nursing staff
and the patient population are constantly changing, and
crucial events such as treatment and discharge are often
quite unpredictable.

It is clear that as development proceeds the child will
become increasingly able to anticipate events and to
construct stable expectations concerning the appropriate
means and ends of social interaction in hospital.   These
anticipatory meanings, however, do not necessarily facilitate
adjustment to hospitalisation;   young children are likely to
focus primarily upon the anticipation of pain and discomfort,
rather than upon the positive functional consequences of
treatment, more remote in time.   Even for the present sample
of older children, differences of educational level were
correlated with differences in the time perspective for
treatment perceptions, and there was evidence that these
factors related to behavioural adjustment in the ward.   The
shift from a concern with immediate consequences towards a
concern with diagnosis and prognosis involves a change to
the validation of meaning at a higher level of cognitive
development.   The locus of uncertainty and conflict will
therefore become increasingly internalised and symbolic as
the child's conceptual environment expands.   In so far as
the complex and ambivalent organisations of meaning
revealed in the conceptions of older children cannot be
effectively constructed, social discontinuity will become
more and more a problem of conceptual discontinuity.   The
standards for validation, and the problems of meaning, will
change and become increasingly orientated towards the future
rather than towards the past or the present.

It is not clear when such time perspectives for validatory
processes will change, nor how much they are dependent upon
social experience or cognitive growth.   However, the effect
of social discontinuity was still found to be important
amongst some of the older girl patients in this study, for
whom a perceived discrepancy between a valued home life and
a disvalued ward life was significantly associated with
reported anxiety behaviour, independent of illness-treatment
conceptions;   this expression of 'value-loss' in social
relationships is suggestive of the separation-distress
frequently found in much younger children, and essentially
reflects a comparison of the experienced present with a
valued and familiar past.   For other children, of course,
there was equally an experience of 'value-gain'.

CONCLUSION

It is evident that much more research is required before one
can speculate further about the function of meaning with
regard to child patients in hospital. Such studies,
however, could lead to a better appreciation of what might
be done to prepare children, both during and prior to
hospitalisation, for the experience of illness and treatment.
They are particularly relevant to the difficult problem of
communication in hospitals. But the present findings
perhaps most of all highlight the immense difficulties
facing practitioners in their everyday attempts to interpret
the behaviour of young patients in their care. The common-
sense vocabulary of motives, which all of us tend to use in
such situations, may refer to 'the naughty child', 'the
awkward child', 'the spoilt child', 'the lazy child', or the
child from a particular 'social class'. Such labels,
however, fail to do justice to the patients' serious
endeavours to find meaning and purpose in their situations,
to establish hope and to overcome fear.

The aim here has been to promote a continued interest in
these theoretical but human problems; it is also intended
to narrow the conceptual gap which has separated studies of
younger children from those of adult patients, by focusing
on a common perspective of meaning from both a socio-
psychological and a developmental viewpoint.

CHAPTER FOUR

The Meaning of Hospital: Denial of Emotions

Ruth Jacobs

INTRODUCTION

Styles of coping with processes of illness and disease in
the West contrast markedly with those characterising other
societies, notably some pre-literate ones where illness and
disease are perceived in ways which take into account an
individual's total social situation and feelings. Thus,
in some cultures both physical and mental sickness are viewed
more holistically than in the West. In such contexts certain
perceptions and explanations of illness may have significant
moral components and as such, may have a powerful role as
mechanisms of social control. Thus, in certain social
contexts illness may be perceived in relation to an
individual's integration into a group. For example, Evans-
Pritchard's classic studies of the Azande (1937) and the
Nuer (1956) both contain detailed analyses of the role that
illness and disease may play within explanatory cosmological
systems, in being associated with aspects of belief systems
which are concerned with 'the particularity of misfortunes'-
why particular persons suffer them (Gluckman, 1965).
    The view of illness and disease as misfortune is one aspect
of a consideration of these phenomena as crisis events.
Illness may be considered as crisis from a variety of view-
points. Such an approach may illuminate certain distinctive
aspects of both individual and group functioning. One reason
for the appeal of this view of illness as crisis is the
inherent contrast such an approach presents in comparison
with the routinised management which characterises many
Western 'caring institutions'.
    In the West illness tends to be viewed within the frame-
work of a model deriving from the natural sciences. Thus,
in general, Western medicine seeks to establish causal
connections between pathological functioning and specific
symptoms. Furthermore, the view of illness within the

framework of a natural-science model has extended to hospitals and to some of those who work in them. Today much of the emphasis in our health-care system tends to be on pathology: combating and responding to illness and disease. We have a 'national *sickness* service' rather than a 'national *health* service'. As part of this process a battery of elaborate technological responses to illness and disease has been devised. Hospitals are part of this specialised provision (Illich, 1975; Foucault, 1973). Furthermore, there has been little emphasis hitherto on encouraging individuals to feel responsible for maintaining and retaining their own health. Indeed, the growing complexity of the social organisations and institutions involved in therapeutic care increases the likelihood that, with the attendant specialisation, people will come into contact with a separate range of functionaries at different points in the illness process. Associated with this complexity is a tendency to detach symptoms from the person manifesting them. This results partly from fragmentation of the illness experience, which has several aspects.

CONSEQUENCES OF THE PROFESSIONALISATION OF HEALTH

In urban industrialised societies such fragmentation is associated with the development of corps of specialists who take over partial or total responsibility for certain major life-events or life-crises - for example, birth, death and illness. Thus, experiences inherent to the human condition are deemed appropriate for specialist control. Similarly, responsibility for certain aspects of sickness and disease is handed over to professionals. Furthermore, in the West the medical professional role is 'functionally specific' (Parsons,1951) - that is, those working as specialists in health and disease are expected to apply their knowledge and skills to problems of illness and the promotion of health and to restrict their professional concern to these areas.

This handing over of areas of care to professional control is a striking characteristic of our society (Schumacher, 1973). The process may apply to either adults or children. However, it is particularly striking in relation to those children who are handed over to the care, influence or control of others. In this way particular aspects of socialisation may be entrusted to specific agencies - for example, schools.

Hospitals further illustrate some of the attitudes to certain life-events and experiences which prevail in industrialised Western societies. Today the word 'hospital' suggests an establishment where sick or wounded people

receive elaborate medical or surgical care. The word has
not always had this meaning: originally the word 'hospitium'
referred not to an institution concerned with disease but
to a place where a guest was received. The hospitalia of
the early Middle Ages were primarily guest houses for
pilgrims (Dubos, 1968). Later the hospital became a place
of detention (Foucault, 1967).

The professionalisation of disease and illness which
characterises Western medicine has inevitably affected the
ways in which these processes are perceived and handled
(Freidson, 1970). In some ways it is consistent with a
fragmented orientation that the feeling dimension of the
illness experience may be neglected or denied. Such an
orientation would be less likely were people perceived more
holistically. However, with the fragmentation of care, the
feelings not only of the patient and his family, but also
of those involved in treating and caring for him, may be
neglected, denied or ignored. This may be part of a
disciplined disregard considered necessary for the detached
and dispassionate scientific diagnosis and treatment of
disease.

THE EFFECTS ON PATIENTS

However, in common with most human experiences, the
processes of becoming and being ill are likely to have
significant affective and psychological dimensions. More
than one hundred years ago (1859) Florence Nightingale was
emphasising these aspects of sickness: 'The least thing can
depress, even alarm, a patient: the nurse's cumbrous dress -
a nurse who rustles is the horror of a patient though
perhaps he does not know why, or sudden jarring sounds -
unnecessary noise is the most cruel absence of care which
can be inflicted.' Moreover, no one should 'make light of
the patient's danger and exaggerate their probabilities
of recovery'.

There is a dialectical interaction between the person as
patient and his symptoms; thus a person may become
dependent, alienated, introverted and cut off because of his
clinical symptoms; he may also regress. The state of being
ill may in itself produce intense feelings, not only in the
patient but also in those who have close relationships with
him, or in those caring for him. How much stronger are these
feelings likely to be when the sick person is a child and
when this child is removed to an unfamiliar environment?

The importance in certain circumstances of the social and
psychological context of illness is now being increasingly
recognised (Zola, 1975a). For example, it is now acknowledged

that a high proportion of long-stay patients remains in
hospital primarily because of the absence or collapse of
a family support system. This factor is particularly
significant in relation to the hospital care both of children
and of elderly people (Stockwell, 1972; Topliss, 1974).

The following case study analyses aspects of the social
relations in a specific hospital and in particular, of one
children's ward within it. This analysis illustrates some
of the values and attitudes that characterise our society.
For example, the study illustrates that there are certain
similarities in social values and attitudes relating to
children and to older people in our society. This is probably
because these two categories of people also have social
characteristics in common: for example, their dependence
and their low social status, which derive partly from the
fact that often they are not permitted to participate
fully in the community as economic agents. In the one case
(older people) this is usually because they have been
compelled to withdraw from this status (Robb, 1967); in
the other (children) it is because they have not yet attained
it. Certain attitudes prevailing within some institutions
reflect such evaluations.

THE CASE-STUDY

The prevailing ideology and value-system of the particular
hospital under consideration illustrate an orientation to
illness and disease which characterises some aspects of
Western medicine today. Within this I suggest that this
particular hospital can be analysed as a partially closed
social system with its own prevailing ideology. I refer
here to Geertz's (1964) analysis of ideologies. He suggests
that as systems of interrelated legitimations, ideologies
give cognitive and normative order to particular aspects of
social reality; they 'name' situations in such a way as to
entail an attitude towards them. Geertz argues that the
construction and use of an ideology is an occurrence not
'in the head' but in the public world where 'people talk
together, name things, make assertions, and, to a degree,
understand each other'. Hence, an ideology is not subject
to standards of scientific rationality but is 'accurate' if
it serves to make sense of action in a particular situation.
Applying Geertz's definition of ideology, I suggest that this
specific hospital was characterised by a prevailing ideology
dominated by the denial, suppression or disapproval of the
overt expression of feelings and emotions.

Thirty-eight child-patients were present in a children's
orthopaedic ward over a five-month period of fieldwork during

which I lived in the hospital.   There were twenty-two beds
in the ward and throughout most of this period they were all
occupied.   The age-range of the children was from six months
to eleven years.   Twenty-six of the total sample were con-
genitally handicapped, with nine suffering multiple
congenital handicap, such as spina bifida or cerebral palsy.
Length of stay in the hospital ránged from a few hours to
several months;   the mean was thirty days.

Certain distinctive characteristics of the patient
population might have countered an ideology characterised by
a denial of feeling, and indeed, might have brought about
an affective and individualistic orientation to the children.
For example, the non-emergency character of much of their
treatment: almost all the children were 'cold' admissions.
In addition, many spent relatively long periods in the ward:
the average length of stay was one month.   Hospital stays
of this length could have been seen as opportunities for
staff and children to establish relatively close relationships with each other.   Moreover, a high proportion of the
children in the ward was re-admissions.   This is an out-
standing characteristic of many children's orthopaedic wards,
reflecting the relatively high incidence of *congenital*
orthopaedic handicap among such children (Pill with Jacobs,
1974).   Some of these children require intermittent hospital
treatment which may extend over many years.   Often the
stages in such treatment relate to bone growth and other
aspects of physical development.   Several children in the
ward had already spent a number of years in this particular
hospital.   It seemed probable that some others were likely
to do so.

For many child orthopaedic patients there are periods
of several weeks, or even months, when their primary medical
need is that certain limb(s) be kept immobilised.   I do not
want to underestimate the significance of this imposed state
of immobility, but suggest that this should not in itself
be identified with clinical illness.   In this context
children's sense of the passage of time is particularly
significant (Goldstein, Freud and Solnit, 1973).

Although these characteristics of the patient population
might have encouraged a personalised, affective orientation
to the children among staff, I suggest that in reality
certain organisational features obstructed and prevented the
development of such a value-system.

ORGANISATIONAL CHARACTERISTICS OF HOSPITAL AND TREATMENT

Certain characteristics of this particular hospital and of
its staff contributed to the creation and maintenance of a

distinctive and predominating value-system. Public transport
facilities were poor and the hospital had a very extensive
catchment area, culling patients from a distance of several
hundred miles. Jones (1975) has pointed out that very often
such institutions are sited a considerable distance from the
nearest towns. Moreover, she writes, 'even hospitals which
are not physically isolated, may share the social isolation
of those that are'. The physical isolation, which was one
way in which this hospital was cut off from the society
beyond its physical boundaries, symbolised the denial of
feeling which took place within it. There was also a notable
absence of certain kinds of links with the world outside
the hospital: for example, there were no social workers
on the hospital staff. I suggest that the relatively closed
character of the hospital as a social system increased the
likelihood that the social organisation within it would be
characterised by a distinctive ideology.

The maintenance and stability of a predominant value-
system within the hospital was also related to the low staff
turnover, particularly among the most senior and the most
junior staff. For example, a very high proportion of the
ward Sisters had been trained in this particular hospital.
(I was told that 15 out of 18 of the Sisters had trained there.)
Many of the auxiliary nurses and domestic staff had worked
in the hospital for several years. Some of them lived
relatively locally and the working hours in the hospital
suited them, often corresponding with their husbands' shift
work. Some staff who had worked in the hospital over a long
period expressed feelings of loyalty to a particular ward,
and resented being moved to another. This stability among
certain categories of ward staff increased the likelihood
that a distinctive ideology, once established, would persist;
such people could act as culture bearers in the ward.

Within the hospital the predominating ideology of a denial
of feeling was reflected in the variety of ways in which ward
staff were fragmented (Miller and Rice, 1967). Various
aspects of the social structure and organisation of the
ward perpetuated this lack of integration among the ward
staff. Certain categories of staff had little contact with
each other, and there were no opportunities for all the staff
involved in a child's care to discuss his welfare together.
There were no case conferences.

The rigid hierarchical structure within the hospital
organisation blocked communication about patients between
different categories of staff. The very complexity of the
hospital structure constituted a social system comprising
at least three major hierarchies: nursing, medical and
administrative. In general, the more people and levels
involved in communication, the more difficult it is to

ensure the free flow of information. One way in which
potentially antagonistic categories of staff prevented open
conflict was through mutual avoidance. Consequently,
confrontations in terms of precedence were rare; for example
nursing activities were reduced while teachers were in the
ward.

The status boundaries associated with particular roles
also extended to individuals' lives off-duty. With many
grades of staff under the same roof, the rigid hierarchical
structure of formal role relationships correlated with
relationships of avoidance between certain categories of
hospital staff in the informal structure. Thus, off-duty
and away from the ward, informal interaction occurred mainly
between individuals of the same status grade, that is
between peers - for example, student nurses and Sisters.
Perhaps the most uninhibited expression of feelings took
place between people of the same status category (MacGuire,
1968).

SOCIAL STATUS AND ECOLOGY

The fragmentation of the ward staff was also reflected in
the ecological order within the hospital, which itself
sustained the social order. Thus the likelihood of contact
between certain grades of staff was reduced by certain featur
of the hospital complex. This is characteristic of total
institutions (Goffman, 1961). Territorial restrictions on
who could go where emphasised such demarcations. Thus within
the hospital complex certain facilities and amenities for
different categories of staff, such as canteen facilities,
were separated.

Status boundaries extended to the location of living
accommodation on the hospital site. The residential
accommodation of different categories of hospital staff
was located in discrete but adjacent zones. In this way
the possibility of chance encounters with other status
categories when individuals were out of their work roles
was reduced. Thus, there were well-defined 'back-stage
areas' (Goffman, 1971) where staff could relax.

The status of various categories of staff was expressed
symbolically in terms of the distance of their residential
accommodation from the locus of the hospital's activity,
that is from the wards. Thus:

Zone 1: *Student nurses* were accommodated in a nurses'
wing within the main block of the hospital complex (that
is, under the same roof). All student nurses were
resident in the hospital for part of their training.
Registrars, who had to be within easy access of the
wards for emergency calls, were also within the main

block but in a separate quarter of the residential part
of the hospital.
Zone 2: *Unmarried senior nursing staff - Matrons,
Sisters and staff nurses* - had residential quarters away
from the main hospital block, in single-storey flatlets.
Some also had their own accommodation away from the
hospital site. For example, a Sister of one of the
children's wards would sometimes go home to her flat,
twelve miles away from the hospital, even if she only
had two hours off duty. She said that she found these
breaks from the hospital environment worth while and
refreshing. (Similarly, many student nurses spent much
of their off-duty time away from the hospital.) This
behaviour illustrated individuals' need for privacy in
the face of the predominantly 'public' social environment which characterises total institutions (Miller and
Gwynne, 1972).
Zone 3: *Senior Registrars* were allocated flats which
were even further away from 'the action' of the hospital
itself - that is, the wards. They also had certain
facilities for their families - for example, a crêche
for their children.
Zone 4: *Consultants* had no residential accommodation.
The time which they spent in the hospital was sessionally
allocated.
It can be seen from this that within the hospital hierarchy
the lower an individual's status, the nearer was that
individual to the wards and the more time did he/she spend
within the hospital. Conversely, the higher an individual's
status in the hospital hierarchy, the less time was spent
there.

CATEGORISATION OF PATIENTS AND DENIAL OF THEIR INDIVIDUALITY

Distinctive characteristics of certain orthopaedic conditions
may have fostered a depersonalised orientation in staff to
their child patients. One factor which may be relevant
here is the inappropriateness to many orthopaedic cases of
the orthodox model of a cure. When patients get better it
is a most reassuring event for their doctor or nurse;
cured patients do great service to their therapists and
nurses (Main, 1968). The best kind of patient for this
purpose is one who, from great suffering and from being in
danger of losing life or sanity, responds quickly to a
treatment that interests the doctor, and thereafter remains
completely well. In a number of ways orthopaedic care and
treatment may not always conform to this ideal.
    Thus certain orthopaedic treatments necessarily extend

over long periods - sometimes years. Moreover, the final
result may not always constitute a 'cure' in the conventional sense; for example, a child may be left with a
residual handicap. This was certainly the situation for
many children in the particular hospital in question. In
medical terms those who recover slowly or incompletely are
less satisfying. The significance of doubt and uncertainty
for medical staff in the performance of their role has been
analysed by Fox (1975). With patients who do not get
better, or who even get worse in spite of long, devoted
care, major strain may arise. Those who attend the patient
are then pleased neither with the patient nor with themselves, and the quality of their concern for him alters
accordingly, with consequences that can be severe for both
patient and attendants (Main, 1968). A similar situation
characterises geriatric medicine: medical staff cannot
'cure' elderly people of old age. Moreover, in the hospital
under study the very fact that many children return
repeatedly for further treatment may itself be a source of
discomfort and dissatisfaction to medical and nursing staff.
These children are symbolic reminders to staff that their
work is incomplete and may not always be totally successful.

The notion that social structures not only provide means
through which a specific task is performed but also equip
members with defences against anxiety is now well established
(Jaques, 1956; Menzies, 1960; Bion, 1961; Coombs and
Goldman, 1973). Menzies in particular has demonstrated how
the social structure of a hospital is used by nurses as a
defence against the anxieties of their job that arise from
the problems of providing intimate physical care and from
their encounters with death. In the particular hospital
being studied the prevailing ideology of denial of feeling
served as just such a coping mechanism.

Ways in which ward staff perceived the children in the
ward, illustrated one dimension of this ideology. Many
staff had a very distinctive perception of the children in
the ward. This related to their categorisation and classification of these children primarily as patients and, moreover
as patients of a particular kind. This view of the children
derived partly from depersonalisation processes which
transformed or converted the child into a patient.

Depersonalisation processes represented aspects of an
ideology concerned with the denial of feeling. Depersonalisation distanced people from one another and therefore
lessened the likelihood of empathy between them. Empathy
is a reciprocal identification process which may act as a
safeguard against depersonalisation. By depersonalising
situations, individuals may attempt to insulate themselves
from the hurt they may themselves be caused by inflicting

suffering on others. Thus, the 'clinical detachment'
(Menzies, 1960; Coombs and Goldman, 1973) apparent in the
attitudes of some hospital staff may be considered a defence
mechanism.
    Parsons's (1951) dichotomy of an affective-instrumental
orientation is relevant here. Parsons suggested that those
concerned professionally with health and disease are expected
to be objective and emotionally detached in their interaction
with patients. Although this model has frequently been
challenged - for example, by Bloor and Horobin (1975) and
by Freidson (1975), who stress certain tensions in the
doctor/patient relationship - nevertheless these concepts
may be useful heuristic devices. In fact, values and
attitudes typifying many staff in this particular hospital
seem to constitute an orientation to the child patients
which was predominantly instrumental in character. Indeed,
because certain staff perceived the children in the ward in
terms of a number of fragmented dimensions rather than
holistically, it was highly probable that such staff would,
in fact, relate to them instrumentally.

DEPERSONALISATION AND 'RITES DE PASSAGE'

The processes by which a child became a patient constituted
a 'rite de passage' - a transition ritual which punctuated
this change in a child's status. In analysing 'rites de
passage' van Gennep (1960) identified three distinctive
stages in these transformations in status. Thus, *rites of
separation* involve stripping a person of certain aspects
of a former identity. For example, there were severe
restrictions on the property and possessions children could
bring with them into the hospital. Children were permitted
to bring only one toy. The admission procedure can also be
regarded as a marginal rite. Among other things this
involved a senior nurse taking personal and medical details
about the child from the parents when they brought him/her
into hospital. A senior nurse also personally introduced
the newly arrived child to each of the other patients in
the ward. *Marginal rites* represent an intermediary stage
comprising the process of elision. This was represented by
the 'waiting period' prior to the beginning of treatment.
Sometimes children were admitted more than a week before
operation. *Rites of aggregation* is the third stage and
involves the creation of the 'new' identity. In this
particular hospital, these rites involved establishing the
identity the patient had while he was in hospital - that of
a hospital patient to whom staff would, on the whole,
relate in an instrumental way.

Following these 'rites de passage' children emerged with a new identity and were objectified in certain ways by some ward staff. One characteristic of the depersonalisation processes associated with transforming the child into a patient was that they enabled staff to perceive and relate to the child in terms of a variety of fragmented dimensions. It follows that having fragmented the child's identity, many staff did not relate to the child holistically. Furthermore, they considered the child's techno-physical needs as primary.

These classification and categorisation processes de-emphasised and ultimately denied a child's individuality - that is, they were concerned with the destruction of his unique identity. I suggest that children's individualistic characteristics threatened to undermine the capacity of staff to sustain and maintain an ideology characterised by the denial of feeling. Awareness of individuality could have led staff towards a realisation of children's unique and individual needs. Such an orientation was antithetical to the prevailing ideology within the hospital. It could also have made the performance of certain activities and procedures by staff more painful and difficult for them (Miller and Gwynne, 1972; Davies, 1976).

DENIAL OF INDIVIDUALITY AND DENIAL OF FEELING

Feelings and emotions are one way in which individuality is manifested. It was logical, therefore, that a denial of individuality should correlate with a denial of feeling. Furthermore, because the expression of particular forms of feeling has to be individualised, it follows that because individuality was denied, so was effect. Certain kinds of affect derive from an awareness and appreciation of individual qualities and characteristics and are therefore incompatible with a collective orientation. It was consistent with this that many ward staff were preoccupied with the needs common to *all* the child patients - their techno-physical needs. Psycho-social needs were underplayed, if not ignored.

How was this achieved? One means was through treating the children as objects. An aspect of this process involved perceiving and classifying the children on the basis of general properties and characteristics; for example, on the basis of certain diagnostic criteria. The more pre-valent was this process of generalisation and abstraction, the more likely was it that this environment would be characterised by a denial of feeling.

While they were patients, the children in the ward were depersonalised in various ways. For example, staff attempted

to equalise and 'level out' the children, thereby disguising
their individuality. This is the 'block treatment'
(Goffman, 1961) common in certain total institutions. For
example, grouping together this heterogeneous category of
children, whose ages ranged from 6 months to 11 years,
indicates that in some ways at least, they were similarly
classified. This form of social organisation also relates
to certain aspects of the ideology of nursing. For example,
nurses are trained to apply a principle of 'fairness' to
patients, not to discriminate between them and to respond
to people and situations with 'detached concern' (Merton
et al., 1957; Towell, 1975). This represents a further
dimension of the denial of individuality which characterises
some institutions.

Moreover, there was a tendency among some staff to consider
a child's current stay in hospital as an isolated episode
in the present, separate from his past and future (Roth,
1963; Ornstein, 1969). The predominant orientation was
not processual or longitudinal. Generally, staff did not
view this particular hospital stay in the context of a
child's wider life experience. Thus staff made little or no
attempt to interrelate sequential aspects of children's
experience - for example, to view this stay in relation to
others, either in the past or in the future. This was one
way staff depersonalised children. The ward-admissions book
illustrated their approach: there was no way of readily
identifying from this record whether children had been in
hospital before. In fact, re-admitted children comprised a
high proportion of the ward intake.

This orientation, which was adopted by some hospital
staff, can be regarded in part as a defence mechanism. By
relating to a child's *current* clinical condition they
distanced themselves from considering the total impact of
certain experiences, both on the child and on his family
(Menzies, 1960). Those in the medical role are exposed to
death, pain and suffering, yet they are expected to respond
with reason and restrained emotionality. The denial of
feeling can be regarded as a coping mechanism which resolved
this dilemma to some extent (Coombs and Goldman, 1973).
This orientation permitted staff to continue their work
without too painful personal distress about the frustration
of their therapeutic wishes (Main, 1968). However, such an
approach increased the likelihood that the child's psycho-
social needs in the hospital could be neglected or ignored.

The denial of feeling is illustrated further by the
general reluctance to acknowledge that certain activities
and procedures could have disturbing effects on children.
Thus, there was no systematic policy of preparation for
forthcoming treatment procedures. In general the ward was

an environment in which things were *done to* children,
without their necessarily understanding what was going on,
and with little attempt to involve them in these procedures.
Indeed, it appeared that for some staff the ideal was for the
children to be passive objects.

SOCIAL ORGANISATION OF THE WARD AS A BARRIER TO PERSONAL SOCIAL RELATIONS

The social organisation of the ward worked against the
formation and growth of relationships between individual
staff and specific children. The fragmentation of the
children's care referred to earlier illustrates this point.
Both the hospital and the ward itself were run in ways that
prevented staff from forming and maintaining close relationships with patients.

The lack of continuity in ward staff was one factor that
was significant in preventing the development of personalised
relationships between staff and children. For example,
doctors were rarely in the ward and generally children
could only have tenuous links with them (MacCarthy, 1974).
Of senior nursing staff, the ward Sister was probably the
person most continuously present. Auxiliary and domestic
nursing staff were also relatively stable elements in the
composition of the staff. However, there was no practice
of patient assignment in this hospital. Staff nurses
changed fairly regularly. Each student nurse was in the
ward for a maximum of only six weeks. The implications
of such breaches in continuity among those caring for
children have been extensively investigated (Goldstein,
Freud and Solnit, 1973; Clarke and Clarke, 1976; see also
Brown, ch.2).

Hospital school staff were in the ward for relatively
short periods on weekdays during school terms. They were
away from the hospital at weekends and throughout school
holidays. Thus a child could pass the whole of his stay in
hospital without seeing a hospital teacher at all. Moreover,
while teachers were away from the hospital, school equipment
and toys were locked away, so children could not have
access to them.

We know from activity-sampling data (Pill with Jacobs,
1974) that the category of staff with which children had
most frequent and regular contact - the student nurses -
was that whose composition changed most often. This was
because of factors such as the eight-hour shift system,
the six-weekly turnover of student nurses (which was
related to the structure of their training scheme) and the
special weekend rotas. Such changes in ward staffing would

work against the development of close relationships between
staff and specific children (Towell, 1975). Thus, staff
turnover and the shift system worked against a personalised
affective orientation between ward staff and children. One
consequence of children's dependence on ward staff was that
subsequently such people could control many aspects of
what happened to the children while they were in the hospital.
Staff were active agents in processes which initially deprived
children of initiative, autonomy and choice. Having
classified children primarily as patients, henceforth many
hospital staff related primarily to their techno-physical
needs.

This value-system of staff had implications for *all*
patients in the ward; for example, it was reflected in the
time and attention each was accorded. Priority was given
to clinical activities. Thus staff who were *not* primarily
concerned with the child's *clinical* needs - for example,
teachers, occupational therapists, and certain other
auxiliary staff - were accorded relatively low status
within the ward hierarchy. Furthermore, many children in
this particular ward had 'waiting periods' of several weeks
or even months, while they were in plaster or traction.
During these times their clinical needs were relatively few.
Then they received relatively little regular attention from
ward staff, apart from care for their basic physical needs,
such as toileting and feeding. Indeed, when hospital staff
could no longer bring about significant change in a child's
clinical condition, in effect they wrote the child off, in
terms of the amount of attention given. This was particularly
evident in the case of the two longest-stay children in the
ward, both of whom had degenerative diseases and had been
in the hospital for several years.

BEDFASTNESS AND DEPENDENCY

Some of the processes by which a child was subjected to
hospital control affected the child's physical status in
striking and dramatic ways. For example, most of the
children in the ward were bedfast throughout their stay in
the hospital. It is striking that bedfast people comprise
distinctive social categories, for example, babies, the sick
and some elderly people, all of whom are dependent individuals
generally acknowledged as not having full social status
within the community.

The high proportion of bedfast patients is one of the
most distinctive characteristics of certain children's
orthopaedic wards, although in some of the most advanced
wards every effort is made to make the children mobile.

This hospital was not one of these. Most children were
confined to bed as soon as they arrived in the ward. In a
very real sense, being bedfast transformed a child's identity.
Children were compelled to be horizontal and consequently may
have felt prone and vulnerable. In addition, many were put
into either traction or plaster, their bodies thereby being
transformed and their mobility restricted further.

In confining children to bed, ward staff enforced
dependence upon them in a variety of ways. Bedfastness also
restricted the ways children could affect, influence or
control what was going on around them, or could even find
out about this. Moreover, although staff could easily
initiate contact with children, it was relatively difficult
for children on their part to withdraw from such initiation.
This is a further illustration of the power imbalance
between staff and children (Hall, 1977).

Thus, many children, partly because of their clinical
condition and the physical constraint consequently imposed
on them, were deprived of ways in which they would otherwise
have been able to seek various kinds of stimulation. A
considerable amount of work has been done to investigate
the possible consequences of such deprivation (Pringle,
1964; Winnicott, 1971; Goldstein et al., 1973).

It was consistent with the processes by which children,
on becoming immobile, also became dependent, that as soon
as they were no longer bedfast and dependent in other ways,
they were discharged from the ward - indeed, sometimes even
before their family was really able to cope with the home
situation. Very rarely were there any mobile children in
the ward.

Why was this? One reason may have been a need for beds
in the ward. I was told by the hospital's admissions
secretary that the period of waiting for admission to this
particular ward for cold surgery could be as long as
eighteen months. However, general ward practices did not
always make the most economical use of the beds available -
for example, sometimes children were in the ward for more
than a week before surgery.

I suggest that in fact there may have been other reasons
for discharging children once they were regaining mobility.
For example, such a child was moving towards re-establishing
the identity formerly had outside the hospital. Ward staff
may have perceived this transitional stage as 'dangerous'
in the sense used by Douglas (1966). Once beginning to
regain mobility, a child was re-establishing his/her former
identity. In the ward a mobile child represented a potentially
undisciplined force that staff might not be able to control.

CONSTRAINTS ON CHILDREN'S BEHAVIOUR

It was not only the children's *physical* state that was
constrained and restricted in the ward: their behaviour
was also circumscribed in certain ways. Thus attempts were
made to induce children to behave in approved ways. The
corollary of this was that staff attempted to diminish or
extinguish certain responses in the children if such
responses were troublesome for them; for example, drugs
were sometimes used as a means of controlling children. We
have observational evidence that staff judging a child to
be particularly obstreperous or difficult to handle might
give the child a tranquillising drug.

I suggest that in certain circumstances these responses
and reactions from the children - for example, depression or
mild hysteria - were *normal* reactions to pathological or
abnormal situations. Thus (Veeneklaas, 1976):

Separation depression is a phenomenon prevalent in all
living individuals. It is caused by deprivation of the
trusted home environment. It is neutralised by reunion
with that home. In the paediatric setting we meet the
phenomenon regularly in children, aged 1-4, who have to
be admitted and are by that process deprived of their
homes, in which the mother acts as the living centre.

One effect of the 'environmental press' (Tizard, Sinclair
and Clarke, 1975) of this hospital organisation was that
instead of modifying the caring environment to meet patients'
needs, attempts were made to bring about their adjustment
to this situation. The result of this was that the hospital
environment itself remained relatively unchanged. The
social environment of the hospital was not responsive to
individual, or even group, needs.

Because patients were considered primarily in terms of
their techno-physical needs, when a child required little
'technical' nursing, he received little attention from ward
staff. One way a child could get attention from ward staff,
however, was by actively seeking it by asserting her/himself
in the ward situation. However, the mode of behaviour
approved by staff was for a child to be obedient, quiet
and unobtrusive. This view favoured the creation of an
environment which might repress and suppress some of a
child's spontaneous reactions to the ward environment.
There were no direct outlets in the ward situation for a
child's fears and anxieties about hospital and his/her
illness. The value and importance of taking account of
children's own feelings about various aspects of their
illness experience is now well established (Gordon, 1974).
The response of some children to this environment was withdrawal and depression. It was particularly unfortunate that

this response conforms with some nurses' concept of 'the good patient' (Hawthorn, 1974; Lorber, 1975).

The ward was a deprived environment in terms of the general absence of stimulation for children. There was little to engage their sustained interest and attention. Furthermore, the lack of individualised contact with staff in the ward, together with the general atmosphere of noise and activity, was likely to prevent or at least disturb children's concentration. The close proximity of beds, the large number of under-fives in the ward during this period, and the consequent possibility of interruptions and distractions from children in neighbouring beds, added to their problems. It could be difficult for children to occupy themselves independently - for example, in reading or other solitary activities. In this situation children readily turned to seeking attention from staff. To some extent they had succeeded if they managed to do merely this, regardless of whether this attention took the form of positive or negative sanctions.

ROUTINE AS A BARRIER

The ward routine further illustrated depersonalisation processes. Patients were subjected to rigid ward routines which treated all children similarly, thereby ignoring their individuality. Much of this ward routine focused on aspects of the children's physical condition. This rigid routine dominated hospital life (Davies, 1976). Through the ward routine staff asserted one dimension of their control of the ward environment.

Such routine procedures implicitly denied the individuality of *both* staff *and* patients, subjecting all patients to the same procedures and thereby de-individualising them. Thus, one effect of the 'environmental press' was to induce conformity, stamping on to all the child patients a similar institutional imprint. The ward regime left children little or no opportunity to exercise choice or initiative. Thus this institution was concerned with transforming the children into passive receptors rather than responding to them in terms of their own unique experiences and needs. This tendency is in the reverse direction of socialisation processes which are generally concerned with encouraging the child to be independent and autonomous (Wheeler, 1966). The hospital system worked in the direction of depriving the children of initiative, autonomy and choice.

It was consistent with this that many nursing staff did not consider social contact with the children to be part of their ward work. In fact, they perceived such work

specifically in terms of children's techno-physical needs.
For example, student nurses seen chatting or playing with
children in the ward were sometimes chided by senior nurses
and told to 'get on with their work'.   Similarly, remarks
made by student nurses while watching play-backs of video-
taped material of ward activities clearly indicated that
they did not feel that predominantly *social* interaction
with children was part of their ward work.

The 'busy-ness' of the repetitive routine activities
helped to ensure that staff had little time for spontaneous
contact or communication with patients.   Furthermore,
certain aspects of the ideology of orthopaedic
nursing emphasised this preoccupation with external reality.
Thus in speaking about their work nursing staff stressed
the extreme importance in orthopaedic nursing of continuous
attention to detail – for example, observation of a child's
hair, skin and nails as valuable indices of the child's
general state of health.

All this interest and activity associated with aspects
of external reality deflected attention away from 'internal'
dramas – that is, from the feelings and emotions of those in
the ward (Menzies, 1960).   The regular and repetitive
activities comprising the ward routine also reduced the
visibility and apparent significance of individualistic
activities in the ward.

Some of the effects of routinisation on both patients
and nursing staff have been analysed by Brown (1973).   He
suggests that in routinising jobs there is a danger not only
that the activities will be less well done but that 'the
encumbering routines may well lessen an individual's
chance of developing a perspective and commitment of his
own to the job'.   To counter this, Brown suggests that
'where possible work should be arranged so that non-routine
activities play an important if not dominant role'.

ROUTINE AND THE STEREOTYPED RESPONSE

Some categories of staff, notably student nurses, were
trained to carry out aspects of their work in routine and
functional ways.   Such staff were denied opportunities to
use their creativity spontaneously.   Thus many responses in
the ward situation were relatively stereotyped.   It is
consistent with this that outsiders to hospitals sometimes
comment that in hospitals it is very often ancillary staff
such as hospital porters, ward orderlies and ambulance men
who are most helpful and understanding in their attitudes
towards them.

Why should this be so?   Part of the explanation may be

that appeals for help are unlikely to occur sufficiently
regularly or frequently for response to them to be considered
part of the work of specific hospital staff. That this was
indeed the situation is illustrated by the observation that
in such instances there was no obvious person from whom
help could be sought. It also seems likely that such
incidents were not considered sufficiently important or
significant by hospital staff themselves to merit a worked-
out response. In unfamiliar situations individuals cannot
fall back on stereotyped responses. Therefore, when
approached for help, ancillary staff responded spontaneously
and in a manner which accorded with their own personalities.
It may also be significant that such ancillary staff as
porters, orderlies and ambulance men were not themselves
directly involved in those clinical treatment processes which
might necessarily involve inflicting pain. Therefore
they had less need to distance themselves defensively through
'clinical detachment' from patients and their families.

These points have wider implications: repetitive and
predictable tasks may be associated with rigid and routine
responses, which can themselves depress an individual's
capacity to respond spontaneously and creatively. Moreover
in the circumstances quoted the people concerned were
appealed to as *individuals*. One implication of this is
that collective responsibility, and the submerging of
individual identity which may be associated with it, may
dampen individuals' sensitivity and initiative. These
points are also relevant to a consideration of those hospital
staff who didn't adhere to the prevailing ideology in their
values and attitudes. Thus although the dominant ideology
among hospital staff was concerned with the denial of
feeling, there were some notable exceptions.

It was striking that those highly trained staff whose
orientation to the child patients was relatively individualistic, expressive and affective in character, were people
not working as members of a group or category, but as
individuals - for example, a Sister, teacher and nursery nurse.
Thus they were all people in *singular* role situations.
The autonomy associated with these roles may have led such
individuals to feel personally and individually committed
to, and directly responsible for, the child patients in
their care. The autonomy associated with these particular
roles enabled those occupying them to use their creativity
in the ward situation. Such people felt personally
accountable for their actions in the ward in a way that those
working as one of a category - for example, certain grades
of nurses - may not. Those who work in the ward as one
of a category may be relatively more likely to feel alienated
from their work situation.

EXCLUSION OF OUTSIDERS AS A MEANS OF MAINTAINING IDEOLOGY

The ways in which the hospital's ideology was maintained
illustrated certain other aspects of the relationship
between staff and those outside the social system of the
hospital - in particular, the children's parents. How did
ward staff cope with outsiders to the hospital? How were
children's links to them handled while they were in the ward?
Some staff discouraged the children from activities, forms
of contact or behaviour which could serve to differentiate
between them and thereby emphasise their individuality. The
links that most children had with their homes and families
were one way that this individuality could be expressed.
Thus the severe restrictions on visiting hours and on the
possessions children could bring with them into the ward
were one way in which these ties to the outside world were
controlled, if not actually severed.

Ways in which control was exercised over who could come
into the ward, when, and what they could do while they were
in it, illustrated how staff maintained their distinctive
value-system within the context of their relationships with
those outside the social system of the hospital - and in
particular with children's parents. We have seen that one
way in which the hospital's value-system was maintained was
that, on becoming a patient, the child was subjected to
control by ward staff. One aspect of this process was that
the rival sources of control were discouraged from penetrat-
ing the hospital system.

Some ward staff seem to have viewed the hospital as a
closed system. The extent to which for some children this
particular hospital was indeed an almost totally closed
social system is seen in the situation of those long-stay
children who had lost virtually all contact not only with
their homes and families but also with the outside world
(Oswin, 1971). However, a model of the hospital as a closed
system denies certain aspects of reality - for example,
that a child's stay in hospital is part of an on-going
process and that for most children such a stay necessarily
involves people outside the hospital system. In fact the
boundary of the hospital as a social system can be visualised
as a semi-permeable membrane through which individuals had
to pass in order to enter the hospital. Outsiders could
only gain access through hospital sponsorship: that is,
access was controlled, though it was the children who
legitimated their parent's access. The isolation and
inaccessability of the hospital is likely in itself to
have deterred some potential visitors (Cross and Turner,
1974).

A variety of social control mechanisms regulated contact

between outsiders and the hospital. General hospital policy
was to restrict outsiders' access to the ward. Visiting
hours were strictly circumscribed (Pill with Jacobs, 1974;
Deliege and Leroy, 1976). Furthermore, there was little
provision for outsiders' needs in the hospital: for example,
there were no special facilities for parents as visitors.
Apart from Saturday and Sunday afternoons, when the Red
Cross voluntary group ran a canteen, visitors could not even
get a cup of tea. Thus, although ward staff could not
entirely prevent parents from coming into the ward, they
could restrict their access to it and could influence
factors affecting how parents and others felt while they
were in the ward - for example, whether they felt welcome
or not, how easy it was for parents to cope with their
other children while they were visiting, giving them information about financial assistance with visiting and so on.

Many parents had to spend as long as half a day travelling
from home to the hospital and there were no facilities for
them to stay overnight. Moreover, the categories of permitted visitors were severely restricted: no sibs or other
children were allowed in the children's ward; nor was there
a crêche or anywhere else for them to go while their parents
were visiting in the ward. The rationalisation which was
frequently given for excluding sibs and other children from
the ward was the risk of cross-infection that they constituted. This view is now seriously questioned. Perhaps one
reason for this attitude to other children coming into the
ward related to the fact that child visitors could be
difficult for staff to control. Furthermore, certain staff
may have perceived such children as threatening to their
view of 'the child in hospital'. Thus patients' sibs were
walking reminders of the normal world of childhood outside
the hospital. Therefore they were a symbolic bridge between
the hospital and this outside world. Because of this they
threatened the perception of the hospital as a closed
system.

A further aspect of the control exercised over outsiders
was apparent in the restrictions on what they could do while
in the ward. In fact little attempt was made by hospital
staff to involve parents in ward life while they were
visiting their child. This was despite the fact that many
parents went daily to the hospital over a period of several
weeks, if not months, and therefore must have become familiar
figures in the ward to some staff.

However, one implication of sharing children's care with
their parents would have been that some staff would have
had to adopt an individualistic orientation to each child
and that child's family, taking into consideration many
aspects of their own particular situation. However, ways

in which the hospital was organised encouraged staff to perceive the child patients in terms of *general* categories. In view of this, it was unlikely that staff would think in terms of how the needs of *individual* child patients and their families could best be met. Thus parents and other outsiders to the hospital system met with varying degrees of staff opposition - from indifference to antagonism and hostility.

Why was this? Parents and other outsiders represented the world outside the hospital and as such may have been disquieting symbols to the ward staff. Another source of this ambivalence or hostility may have been that by their very presence parents served to remind staff of the child's socio-emotional needs. Indeed, through being in the ward parents expressed their bond with their own particular child. It was consistent with an emphasis on children's techno-physical needs that those individuals who symbolised the affective dimension of the child's identity were not integrated within the social system of the ward. Thus outsiders such as parents represented different and con-flicting ideologies and value-systems (Voysey, 1975) compared with those characterising the ward. They could be perceived as potential threats to the control that staff exercised in the ward. Moreover, such people were rival sources for control of the child and therefore were potential threats to the status quo. Parents and others represented a source of possible disruption that was beyond the legiti-mate control of ward staff.

Furthermore, parents might transmit or convey emotion into the ward. For example, sometimes one apparent effect of parents' visits was to upset the child. After they left, the child might become distressed and require staff time and attention in being settled. Some staff may have attributed this distress directly to the child's parents. The overt expression of feelings and emotions was anti-thetical to the ethos of this ward and, in so far as staff might perceive that parents could contribute to such expression, they met with ambivalence, if not hostility, in the ward situation. Restricting the access of such people who were beyond the direct authority of the hospital was one way in which the open expression of feelings in the ward was curbed.

INFORMATION CONTROL

As well as avoiding direct contact with parents, one powerful means of social control exercised by staff was to withhold information from parents about what was going on

concerning the patient. The information given to parents
and patients was deficient in both quality and in quantity.
Often contact between the hospital and the child's home
was unsatisfactory and unreliable - for example, communication about admission dates or operation dates. Moreover,
there were no social workers in this particular hospital
at this time. Social workers could have been one means
by which links between home and hospital could have been
established and maintained.

Thus staff exercised their power in the ward by keeping
outsiders in ignorance of what was happening. Lack of
information and knowledge may deprive people of the freedom
to make choices. The various ways in which inadequate
communication between hospital, patient and family may
increase stress and anxiety have been analysed by Harrisson
(1974). Others have suggested that this breakdown in
information flow may actually impede the healing process
(Cassee, 1975).

Although ward staff could not prevent parents from coming
into the ward during the established visiting periods, to
some extent they were able to minimise the amount of direct
contact between themselves and children's parents which
then took place. Generally ward staff were conspicuous by
their absence during visiting times. Indeed, the ward
Sister once said, 'I'll be honest with you: I don't like
parents but I talk to them all every day and I am around
so they can see me.' In fact it was noticeable that she
tended to stay in her office during these periods. Though
theoretically available to parents, they would have
specifically to seek her out to talk with her. Thus the
initiative for such contact with the ward Sister would have
to come from parents themselves. For many, this was
probably a sufficient deterrent to prevent such interaction.
Playing for time was another controlling strategy staff
sometimes employed if parents requested information or
action from them. In fact many parents relied on each other
for information about ward procedures and courses of
treatment. When they did ask ward staff about these
subjects, their questions tended to be directed towards the
least intimidating members of staff - often to domestics,
nursing auxiliaries and, also, to the research worker!

THE PEER GROUP

Although ward staff could apply a variety of positive and
negative sanctions to impose, enforce and maintain the
social order and exercise control over their patients,
nevertheless the children were themselves also able to

influence certain aspects of ward life: for example, they could make things easier or more difficult for staff. To some extent children's power in this situation related to their individual skills and knowledge of the ward as a social system; but, more importantly, the children's capacity to influence ward events derived from their ability to act collectively.

The role of the re-admitted and long-stay children could be particularly critical here. These children, 'the wise' (Goffman, 1963), knew the ropes concerning ward life and activities. They were aware of ways in which they themselves could affect these. In view of the high turnover among some categories of staff, especially night staff, this was particularly significant. Indeed, it is probable that some children knew considerably more about certain aspects of the dynamics of ward life than did many ward staff. This situation endowed specific children with an important role as culture bearers. They could transmit to other children certain kinds of information about how to work the ward system: for example, information about aspects of ward organisation, about ways certain staff could be provoked or taken advantage of by calling for bedpans, urine-bottles or drinks, and so on. To some extent the children's power in this situation was related to the extent of their awareness of this collective strength.

As well as being leaders in this way, individual children sometimes established a group-following by behaving in particular ways, such as calling out, shouting, screaming or crying. We have observational evidence that on some occasions such behaviour was readily taken up by other children - there were several instances of 'evening uproars'. On these occasions older children initially took advantage of the fact that there were few staff in the ward to make excessive demands on staff by calling out for drinks and bedpans. Younger children swiftly followed their example. On one occasion this led to chaos: the only nurse present fled from the ward. Eventually such behaviour inevitably brought attention from staff. Within the context of the ward as a socially deprived environment this may well have been part of what the children were seeking.

Because patients were considered primarily in terms of their techno-physical needs, when a child required little technical nursing, little staff attention was received. Furthermore, the mode of behaviour most approved by staff was for children to be obedient, quiet and unobtrusive. This view favoured the creation of an environment which might repress and suppress some of a child's spontaneous reactions. There were no direct outlets in the ward situation for children's fears and anxieties; nor indeed

were there any ways staff could express feelings of this
kind. Given that the children in general were not able to
establish stable, on-going relationships with members of
the ward staff, what outlets did a child in the ward have for
the expression of feelings and emotions?

I suggest that while they were in the hospital it was
primarily in their relationships with other children, and
in particular in aspects of their play, that some children
liberated and expressed certain feelings and emotions.
How were children's feelings about what was happening to them
in the ward expressed? Sometimes this was in their relationships with other children - for example, in questions, talk
about what would happen to them in the ward, the course of
treatment or operations. This expression was evident in
certain aspects of their play: playing at doctors and
nurses was among the most popular games. Drawing was also
popular among some children.

One of the long-stay 'institutionalised' children
created an elaborate and detailed fantasy world. He spent
considerable periods playing solitary games with himself,
some of which derived partly from the comics he read. Both
he and one of the other institutionalised children had a
very rich fantasy life; they created a world peopled with
a mixture of real and imaginary characters. Many of the
boys in the ward spent a lot of time in aggressive, noisy,
violent play, which often involved the symbolic movement
of toys, or weapons, for example. This could be seen as a
reaction to their own loss of physical mobility.

Many staff seemed to be relatively unaware of the special
significance of the social dimension of children's lives
in the ward. They did not seem to recognise the importance
to children over a certain age of their relationships with
other children. These relationships can help greatly in
making a child's stay in hospital a happier experience.
Alternatively, if things go wrong in the relationships with
other children in the ward, this may upset or worry a child
and may even affect the rate of recovery (Cassee, 1975).
In some orthopaedic wards children's social relationships
with each other are likely to be especially important
because of the long waiting periods associated with
particular treatments. At such times children tended to
have relatively little contact with staff, many of whom
were in any case frequently changing. Moreover, children
had relatively little time with their parents and family
while they were patients in the ward. They had most time
for social contact and interaction with each other. Despite
the patient turnover, other child patients were the most
stable figures in the child's social universe.

When captive in a bed, a child's neighbours in nearby
beds were particularly important and significant to him.

Most children in this particular ward were bedfast for most
of their stay. How patients were allocated to beds therefore was especially important in affecting the potential
structure of children's social relationships in the ward.
Staff had a critical role in influencing this social pattern.

THE HOSPITAL STAFF AS VICTIMS OF THE SYSTEM

Hospital staff were as much victims of an ideology
characterised by the denial of feeling as were the child
patients. The non-supportive character of the hospital
organisation illustrated how this value-system affected
hospital staff as well as patients (Miller and Gwynne, 1972;
Deliege and Leroy, 1976).

Training of some hospital staff neglected certain psycho-
social aspects of their work (Davis, 1975; Towell, 1975).
This in turn had implications for the orientation of staff
within the ward. There appeared to be no organised or
institutionalised means by which staff could legitimately
seek and obtain emotional support in response to psychological and emotional demands made upon them in their work.
For example, some student nurses disliked nursing a battered
child in the ward; indeed, some expressed a strong aversion
to having anything to do with her. Senior nursing staff
seemed to accept this situation, and this particular child
was looked after by those nurses who were willing to care
for her. But this avoidance approach did not help these
young nurses to cope with comparable situations which might
arise for them in the future. It was as if by ignoring
the lack of emotional support the need for it could be
denied.

One could argue that in the ward in question there was
particular need for such support in view of the fact that
the category of ward staff having most frequent and regular
contact with the children were the student nurses, for whom
the experience of working in the ward was a relatively new
one. They were therefore especially vulnerable to the
emotional onslaught of working in a hospital. Many of these
student nurses were only 17 years old. (At this time it
was possible to begin training for orthopaedic nursing one
year earlier than was usual for other branches of nursing.)

One consequence of the lack of support from senior to
junior nurses could have been that student nurses provided
each other with mutual support. Indeed, to some extent
junior nurses *did* form close informal groupings, but in
other respects the social organisation of the hospital
worked against this. Thus student nurses were fragmented
by shift work and the regular changes in the composition
of their work groups.

I suggest that the failure to provide emotional and psychological support to certain staff in the ward had important consequences in terms of the care they themselves were able to give to child patients. Partly because staff were not themselves given support in their own feeling-responses to certain aspects of their work, they were consequently themselves limited in their ability to *give* such support in the ward situation to child patients and their families (Menzies, 1960; Miller and Gwynne, 1972; Cassee, 1975). Some staff responded to such demands either by avoidance or by withdrawal. The fragmented orientation of staff and their preoccupation with children's techno-physical needs increased the likelihood that in the ward situation feelings would be denied or ignored.

CONCLUSION

In common with companion studies in this volume, the implications of the preceding analysis are both theoretical and practical.

My consideration of aspects of the meaning of hospital suggests that to further our theoretical understanding of social processes involved here we need to extend the analytic framework applied to this situation so that it is both more holistic and processual in character. Thus the context within which we look at the illness process should be broadened both in terms of the period of time considered and the extent of the network of roles and relationships involved. Each study within this volume contributes to these ends.

The most important practical implication of the study reported in this chapter emphasises the dialectical character of illness and the social institutions connected with it. Thus in order that staff may themselves provide psycho-social support in the ward situation, both to each other and to patients, they must themselves be given such strength and succour from others within the social organisation in which they work. Furthermore for change to take place within institutions that are dominated by an ideology characterised by denial of feeling, such support must be readily available to staff. This is a necessary pre-condition for change in the orientation of staff. The quality of the care given in the ward will in turn reflect and relate to these values.

CHAPTER FIVE

Demands and Responses
The effects of the style of work allocation
on the distribution of nursing attention

Jean Cleary

OBSERVATION OF CHILDREN'S ACTIVITIES

A study of the effects of introducing a playleader into a
children's ward in a general hospital (Hall and Cleary, 1974;
Hall, 1977) involved extensive periods of observation of
the activities and interactions of the patients, both before
and after the playleader began work. Data were collected,
therefore, which included the movements and actions of nurses
also. It became apparent that the way in which the work of
the nurses was organised had important implications for the
care of child patients.

Within the ward situation some of the work is predictable
- the provision of meals for a known number of patients, for
example - while the rest is variable, dependent upon the
condition of particular patients, like the nature of the
technical nursing procedures to be performed on a particular
day. Nevertheless, if outright emergencies are excluded,
the patients' general needs for nursing and other forms of
physical care can be foreseen and built into a routine which
meets the demands of the situation. In most British hospitals,
including those where the playleader-innovation study took
place, this routine is task oriented. The satisfaction of
emotional and social needs is not so easily planned nor is
it allocated as anyone's duty, and children as patients are
at a disadvantage because they cannot translate their fundamental unease in the strange situation into acceptable
requests which can be met within the routine, nor can they
be reassured by the reasoned appraisal of their circumstances.
They also lack the ability to adapt their physical needs to
comply with the routine of the ward.

Material drawn from activity-sampling (1), which covered
the first week of each of three month-long periods of
in-ward observation, and from the diary records kept by the
observers, can be used to examine the distribution of nursing

attention through the day and the way in which the particular needs, whether articulate or inarticulate, of the children were met. The ward observations reported here lasted from 6.00 a.m. until 11.00 p.m. and I have used the period from 6.30 a.m. to 10.30 p.m., comprising 48 observations.

Patients were admitted with all kinds of conditions, except ENT, eye and infectious diseases, at the rate of about 1,000 a year. The area observed was the open part of the ward, normally containing 22 beds and, after it was opened, the playroom (Figure 5.1).

The open ward could not be observed from outside except through small glass panels in the door, too high to be useful to anyone of medium height. Sister's office was separated from the ward by cubicles and there was no nurses' station in the ward, even at night. We tend to assume that it is primarily from the nurses that the child patient will get cues about expected behaviour in a strange environment and that it is the nurses who will provide for all the child's needs: we find, in a children's book (Ladybird, 1963), the sentence: 'all day and night there are nurses in the ward to look after the patients.' However, during the 16-hour day there were no nurses present in the ward for about 20 of the 48 daily observations, the percentages for the three separate weeks being 40.8 per cent, 42.6 per cent and 45.5 per cent. It must be pointed out that, as Hawthorn (1974) found to be the general case, the children had no means of attracting a nurse's attention other than calling, setting out to look for one or finding someone else - patient or visitor - willing and able to act for them. The very young, the shy, the inarticulate and the bedfast were obviously at a great disadvantage, particularly those ortho-paedic or traumatic cases who were generally put at the far end of the ward, frequently in traction and therefore very much restricted in what they could do for themselves.

AVAILABILITY OF NURSES

DIARY RECORD 1
10.55 a.m. Emma (2½) has dirtied her nappy and keeps calling for help. Staff Beynon passes and says, 'That's right, dear' and goes out of the ward again. Emma then calls to Sandra, who keeps calling until Susan (a cadet nurse) comes, who changes her.

Nurses' attention was not, then, always easily available, but the recorded observations show their appearance in the ward. If the number of nurses recorded as present in the ward ('sightings') is divided by the number of patients, we get a ratio of nurses to patients, and the fluctuation

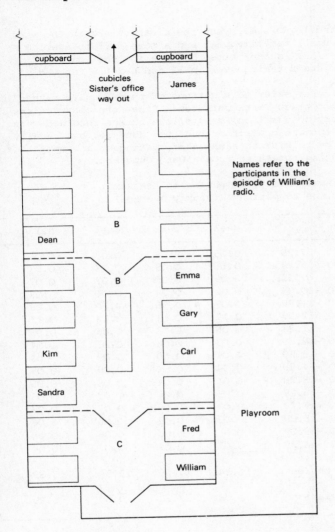

FIGURE 5.1 Sketch plan of the ward

over the day shows the pattern of nursing availability
(Table 5.1). It is at its greatest between 7.30 a.m. and
8.30 a.m., that is breakfast time (which will be slightly
underestimated because one or two children would have been
absent with nurses in the bathrooms), and 11.30 a.m. and
12.30 p.m., that is lunch time, each followed by its toilet
and bed round. The lowest stretch of the day is between

9.30 a.m. and 10.30 a.m., when the cleaners are in the ward. There is a small tea-time peak and a more diffuse evening activity period: supper time, bedtime for the younger ones, night staff taking over, milk and bedtime for the older ones.

These figures refer to sightings of nurses only, rather than actual contacts with children. Since the observations had in theory no duration, many of the nurses recorded were just about to make contact or had just done so, but equally they might be talking to each other, making up an empty bed or fetching something from a ward cupboard.

TABLE 5.1   Availability of nurses in the ward: ratio of nurse-sightings to patients (hourly average)

Hour	Time	Week 1	Week 2	Week 3	All
1	6.30 - 7.29	0.05	0.06	0.08	0.06
2	7.30 - 8.29	0.16	0.09	0.12	0.13
3	8.30 - 9.29	0.09	0.05	0.07	0.07
4	9.30 -10.29	0.02	0.04	0.04	0.03
5	10.30 -11.29	0.07	0.08	0.10	0.08
6	11.30 -12.29	0.17	0.11	0.18	0.15
7	12.30 - 1.29	0.05	0.03	0.06	0.05
8	1.30 - 2.29	0.03	0.06	0.03	0.04
9	2.30 - 3.29	0.09	0.09	0.09	0.09
10	3.30 - 4.29	0.04	0.04	0.09	0.06
11	4.30 - 5.29	0.04	0.04	0.08	0.05
12	5.30 - 6.29	0.05	0.04	0.07	0.05
13	6.30 - 7.29	0.09	0.06	0.07	0.07
14	7.30 - 8.29	0.09	0.03	0.06	0.06
15	8.30 - 9.29	0.03	0.06	0.06	0.05
16	9.30 -10.29	0.05	0.04	0.03	0.04
Mean no. of patients		16.74	17.59	13.34	15.89
Standard deviation		1.03	2.23	0.65	3.89

CONTACTS WITH CHILDREN

The proportions of sightings that were recorded as contacts for the three weeks were 44.4 per cent, 40.4 per cent and 48.2 per cent (average 44.4 per cent). Contacts were divided into two categories, social and nursing, and the latter further broken down into basic and technical.(2) Some contacts fell into both the social and nursing categories, of course, and our interest in this aspect of interaction was stressed to the observers.

TABLE 5.2   Nurse/patient contact as a percentage of sightings

Nature of contact	Week 1	Week 2	Week 3
Social	23.56	29.08	26.35
Nursing	17.29	10.68	17.56
Nursing and social	5.26	2.08	4.82
All contacts	46.12	41.84	48.73
Non-contact sightings	53.88	58.16	51.27
Total sightings	399	337	353

Table 5.2 shows the nature of the observed contacts between nurses and patients. A few contacts would have been missed because they took place behind drawn curtains, which did not allow the observer to code the exchange, but this did not occur more than once a day on average. Neither sightings nor contacts vary directly with the number of patients in the ward. The proportion of contacts which were both social and nursing in content is very low but occurred more often when the nursing was basic rather than technical.

RANGE OF NURSES ON DUTY

The nurses on duty during the early part of the day consisted, typically, of the ward Sister, two staff nurses and a variable number of students, generally between 2 and 6, sometimes a nursery nurse and a nursing cadet. At night there was generally a staff nurse and a student, occasionally a second student or an auxiliary; the latter were seldom seen on the ward. (One or two volunteers usually appeared in the ward at weekends but only one of them, who shortly afterwards began to work in the hospital, made any significant contribution to patient care.)

Qualified nurses accounted for about one-quarter of the total sightings and slightly less of the contacts. Observations showed that they had relatively little purely social contact with the children but that they were more likely to combine social and nursing contact than the students. It may be relevant that nearly all the staff nurses were older women with children of their own.

The ward observations do not tell us the duration of the nursing contact that each child received, but from the case studies (3) we find that for 36 children the average was just under 40 minutes per day (Table 5.3), though there was a wide variation among different children.

TABLE 5.3   Duration of nursing contact

		Mean	S.D.
Month 1	10 cases	54.42 minutes	18.02
Month 2	15 cases	30.06 minutes	17.31
Month 3	11 cases	30.30 minutes	18.20

RESPONSE TO CHILDREN'S NEEDS

These data have shown the way in which the routine of nursing care met the demands of the situation, and consideration will next be given to the adequacy of its response to the particular needs of individual children. Dean Smith of the College of Nursing at the University of Florida has been quoted, in a discussion on the quality of nursing, as saying (in Taylor, 1970):

All patients need to be clean, safe and as comfortable as possible.... The treatment plan of all patients must be implemented. Changes in each patient's condition must be detected and appropriate action based on these changes initiated. The integrity of the therapeutic environment must be maintained.

The picture that emerged from the quantitative studies is of children who were not within sight of a nurse for a considerable part of the day, attention being most reliably available at meal times and the subsequent toilet and bed-making rounds. The way in which this affected the quality of the care provided may now be considered.

The prevailing pattern of available attention was due largely, it seemed, to the organisation of work within the ward; in common with the vast majority of British hospitals a system of task assignment was in use. It is generally agreed that this system tends to produce a task-centred rather than a patient-centred ward and that it increases the number of nurses dealing with each child, which is in itself regarded as undesirable (Ministry of Health, 1959; Hawthorn, 1974). An article in 'Nursing Times', comparing British and American nursing practice, quotes a nurse working on a task-orientated ward: 'I like working here. Sister puts up the work list and we tick off the things as we do them; that way nothing gets missed and you can go off duty happily.' The author comments 'how wrong she was' (Etherington, 1970).

The first factor to stress is that it is apparently the feeling of having satisfactorily completed one's task that encourages the absence of nurses from the ward, for Stockwell (1972) found that 'on the whole when nursing tasks are completed the nurses removed themselves from the patient areas'. Similar tactics were also reported by Dodd (1973). The second factor is the way in which it fragments the nurse's view of a child and prevents her becoming conscious of the unexpressed or inarticulate need, of the   fact that the child who cried during the temperature round is the same one who was crying at breakfast, and crying still rather again. An illustration follows, relating to a boy of nearly 5 with a diagnosis of sub-acute encephalitis, with poor balance and muscle control and unable to speak.

DIARY RECORD 2

6.55 a.m.	Nurse bringing dry pyjamas for James, says to observer: 'Sister is fussy about that.'
7.00	James moans, making noises, lifts head up several times, tries to sit but slips sideways, with head in corner of cot; keeps up noise.
7.10	Nurse 1 passing grimaced at the sight of James.
7.25	James's head still jammed in corner.
7.30	Nurse 2 goes to James but does not shift him.
7.50	Head still jammed.
7.55	Head still jammed.
8.00	Cadet to feed James, does not shift him before she begins.
8.05	She has moved James.

James spent about an hour in a very uncomfortable looking position which he was unable to alter for himself. Admittedly it was a busy time of day but this also meant that there would be nurses in the ward, and his cot was the nearest to the door. The diary record suggests that there would have been at least 17 nurse-sightings during this period, including the serving of breakfast. Two nurses did observe his predicament but did not apparently become conscious of it as something requiring action, perhaps not recalling at the moment that he was incapable of extricating himself from such a position.

This example illustrates another important facet of the task-orientated ward: that when a nurse is in the ward, and therefore potentially available to a child, she is practically always *doing something else*, like the staff nurse quoted in the Diary Record 1.

The substantial absence of nurses, and their frequent preoccupation when present, led to a great dependence on visitors and each other - or at least on the older mobile children: 'Children in traction persuaded other children

to run errands for them...and the service relationship could
on occasions be extended to delivering proxy thumpings or
love letters to the girls' (Hall, 1977). It was not,
however, always the most efficient way of getting things done.

DIARY RECORD 3

7.25 a.m.   (Sandra, aged 12, has sent Kim to find a nurse -
            she had spica plaster put on the day before,
            after nine weeks in traction, and she is
            worried about something.) Ivy (the cleaner)
            sends Kim back into the ward. She complains
            to Sandra, then tries again, waiting until
            Ivy has gone into a cubicle, gets caught
            again and sent back. Sandra sends her again:
            'Say it's important.' Kim says to Ivy 'It's
            important - it's about Sandra's leg'. Mary
            goes to Sandra - Kim got stopped at the first
            cubicle. Staff comes in to fetch something
            from the cupboard and Kim relays Sandra's
            message: 'Sandra's leg's wet.'

Children came to rely upon each other even when nurses
appeared to be available - one recording sheet shows the
following situation: Kim is helping Sandra with a bedpan
and Fred is playing with a baby in a cubicle. Sandra, a
large girl, was in traction at this time, with a broken femur,
and to move such a patient properly requires a skill and
strength unlikely to be deployed by a 7 year old. The
parents of the baby might have been dubious about 12-year
old Fred, who was mentally retarded and had an arm and leg
in plaster. At the time of the recording we can see that
two nurses and the ward receptionist were standing in the
middle of the ward.

I have spoken of the nurses who came into the ward as
having something else to do, being preoccupied, but it
seemed to all the observers that they had developed an
intense concentration on the job in hand, either as part of
their professional training or in sheer defence against the
multiplicity of calls upon them, which was felt to be
inappropriate for a children's ward as in the following
extract:

DIARY RECORD 4

9.04 p.m.   Robert (age 6) with arm in sling, being chased
            wildly round the table by a much larger
            Robert (age 9). Mark (11) joins in and lays
            down chair as an obstacle in small Robert's
            path. Peter (also with fractured arm, age 7)
            climbs on table and dances around. Staff
            nurse comes in with trolley to get something
            from cupboard, does not even glance in the
            direction of children and seems unaware of the
            noise.

It would not be unfair to suggest that the last two incidents showed at least dents in the integrity of the theraputic environment, and some longer examples are now given to demonstrate how these factors can affect the way in which an episode can develop or the care of a 'difficult' child be handled.

THREE EXTENDED EXAMPLES

William's radio (4)

A little before 7.30 in the morning William was sitting up in Gary's bed, and both were listening to the radio that William's parents had given him the day before. He came from the country about 50 miles away and had been specifically instructed by one of the staff nurses not to get involved in fights but in any difficulty to seek the help of a nurse. Gary's home was within a mile of the hospital (and he was confined to bed with instructions to move as little as possible). They were both 9 years old. When William wanted to take his radio away, Gary and Dean, an older boy from the same school, refused to let him. Dean hit William but Gary claimed this as his right and they fought until William broke away. Dean pursued him but stopped when Sandra, the oldest girl in the ward, who was in traction, told him to stop. Gary insisted that the radio was now his, and chanted 'Finders keepers, losers weepers.' William protested, very upset, and Sandra told Gary to give it back; meanwhile Carl, a younger boy who could move and speak only with difficulty, urged William to 'tell', so he approached a staff nurse, but she was just going to leave the ward and did not notice him.

After breakfast, William went back to ask for the radio again and the fighting re-started, in which William was an unwilling participant, but he was getting desperate. Dean egged them on while Sandra attempted unsuccessfully to get another girl to go and stop them. It was now nearly 8.30 and a second staff nurse brought round the washing bowls for the children, and told off the boys, especially William, for behaving as though they were 'in school'. She did not seem to hear his explanations and requests for his radio, and left saying, 'Remember, you're in hospital.' While this was going on Dean ran out and hid it.

After his bath, William searched without result and went back again to ask for the radio. Sandra told them to give it back but when Dean did bring it back later on, he and Gary tossed it back and forth, just out of William's reach. Eventually William grabbed for it, Dean ran off with it

again and Gary twisted William's ear until he cried. The
staff nurse and nursery nurse, apparently undisturbed, were
washing Sandra in her bed nearby during this episode.

Gary now proposed a pillow fight and started to swing
his pillow about, but William kept on asking, 'Where is it?'
and glancing at the two nurses who were now making the next
bed (Emma's) in the hope that they would notice and sort
things out. The staff nurse merely complained at some
length about the quarrellsomeness of boys, stating, 'Girls
are good and never quarrel', which infuriated Gary.
William wandered away.

The first staff nurse now took over the bed-making.
With the nursery nurse she moved on to make Gary's bed and
found the radio in it. He asserted that it was his but
she was doubtful and put it on the table. Carl struggled
to explain to her and when William approached took it to
him. The staff nurse asked whose it was. William said,
'Mine', and she accepted this. The nurses united in con-
demnation of Gary, reciting his past misdeeds and threatening
to tell his mother. It was now 8.50.

In this example several factors had an influence on the
course of events. The incident would not have become so
violent or so prolonged if nurses had been present all the
time or if those who did enter the ward had not been intent
on doing something else. Their fragmented view of the
patients seemed to extend to ignoring clinical considerations
when the behaviour of the boys involved in the fracas was
treated as socially rather than therapeutically undesirable,
perhaps because to the nurses the nursing and social
contexts are almost mutually exclusive; this was borne
out by the small proportion of contacts that fell into
both categories in the activity-sampling. The staff nurse
who told William off for being unruly was the same one who
had instructed him that he must avoid fights. The degree
of disturbance tolerated in the ward was supported by a
stereotype of boys as naturally noisy and aggressive, which
did not fit William at all, being the quiet child of elderly
patients, who suffered extreme distress and anxiety during
this episode.

Distress is the keynote of the other examples, acute
or chronic.

Richard

Richard (aged 4) had been in a cubicle suffering from
concussion but in the evening a child in the open ward
turned out to have an infectious disease and was moved into
the cubicle. Richard's cot was brought into the ward at

8.10 p.m. while he was asleep and just before the night staff came on.

DIARY RECORD 5

9.10 p.m.   Nurse to Richard for blood pressure, etc.
He cries when disturbed, especially for bp.

9.20   Richard starts crying, 'Mammy.'
Fat staff nurse: 'Do you want to wee-wee?'
'No.'
'What are you crying for, then?' 'Mammy.'
'She'll be coming in the morning when it's light.'

9.32   Richard still crying.

9.35   Staff: 'Richard be quiet.'

9.40   Richard, crying more quietly for a little, now gets louder again. Michael (aged 11) calls to Richard, goes to him, offers water - 'No.' Tries to distract him by asking teddy's name, but he just calls 'Mammy' and 'Daddy'. Michael misunderstands - 'Mandy', 'Dandy?' - then realising says, 'Daddy can't come till you've gone to sleep, and I bet you he'll be here when you wake up'.
Staff: 'Daddy will be here in the morning when it's light.' To observer: 'When they're in a cubicle you can shut the door and get a bit of peace.'

9.45   Richard still crying. (No one has explained to him that his bed has been moved from the cubicle while he was asleep; he is looking around anxiously as well as crying.)

9.55   Auxiliary to Richard, she strokes his head. Calming gradually. Staff stands by cot for a moment.

10.00   Auxiliary still stroking Richard. Staff and auxiliary talk to observer about night work: 'We've got three on tonight when it's quiet; would have been glad earlier in the week when we were busy.' Daniel starts making muttering noises, disturbs Michael and Richard, who was nearly asleep. Auxiliary goes to quieten Daniel and Richard starts crying hard again. Michael says: 'Be quiet, Daniel. There's a good boy, you just woke the baby up.'

10.05   Auxiliary leaves Richard and he cries again.

10.20   Staff is with Richard, reminds him that his mother gave him jelly today and he starts to cry for jelly, but when offered jelly he cries 'Mammy' again. Staff says: 'If you don't shut up I'll give you something to cry

for.' Looks a bit sick when she remembers
observer, but says: 'I've tried reason,
now I'll try threats.' Night superintendent
on rounds sits by cot, tries the usual line
about mammy coming tomorrow, talks about
teddy and toy car. Asks Staff if he has been
asleep and just woken up. 'Yes' (in fact just
about an hour). Offers horse but he responds
to everything with 'I want Mammy'.

10.30   Auxiliary back with Richard. He repeats
             continuously, 'I want my Mammy.'

10.35   She leaves him, he clutches the car, crying
             fairly quietly, 'My mammy, my mammy.'

10.40   Richard sits up. Staff comes to look at him,
             does not go close - 'Better if they don't see
             us.' Observer asks if his being moved while
             asleep might have upset him. 'Of course, I
             didn't know that had happened. I wish they
             wouldn't do that. Often a child is worried
             that his mother won't find him when he's
             moved from a cubicle anyway.'

10.50   Richard quiet.

Richard's distress received quite a lot of sympathetic
attention, largely from the auxiliary nurse. This and other
episodes suggest that there is a time limit on reassurance
and comforting (probably varying with the amount of work to
be done) and if the child does not respond satisfactorily
within the time allowed the expressed distress is re-
classified as naughtiness or being spoilt and therefore
undeserving of sympathy. Although the staff nurse agreed
wholeheartedly with the observer's suggestion about the cause
of the distress, Richard had had his chance, because the new
interpretation did not change her attitude nor did she
return to reassure him on the specific point, although he
was still crying.

   Richard, however, got more sympathetic handling than
Judith, the unhappy child in the final illustration. She
was admitted during a period of ward observations and therefore
we have some quantitative measures as well as the diary
record.

Judith (aged 2 years 8 months)

During a period of five days, with a possible total of 211
observations, we get the figures of Table 5.4.

TABLE 5.4 Judith's activities (from activity-sampling)

Observations	Number	%	Number crying	%
Unrecorded	13	6.16	-	-
Asleep	54	25.59	-	-
With parents	36	17.06	4	1.90
With staff	15	7.11	10	4.74
With patients	8	3.79	1	0.47
Alone	85	40.28	46	21.80
Total	211	99.99	61	28.91

DIARY RECORD 6

Evening after admission (5)

6.25 p.m.   Susan rings bell for visitors to leave and
            Judith and Sian scream for mothers not to
            leave the ward. Student nurse collects
            empty supper dishes - takes no notice of
            crying children. Sian's mother talks to
            Judith and says, 'Mummy is coming back now.'
            Judith is inconsolable.

6.42   Judith is still very distressed.

6.50   Staff goes to Judith to change her nappy,
            talks to her, but child is still very
            distressed. Staff says, 'There's a good girl'
            several times.

7.20   Judith still crying bitterly alone.

7.39   Judith has stopped crying - playing with toy -
            starts crying again. Student nurse calls her.

7.44   Judith still crying for her mother.

Judith's fourth day in the ward

6.30 a.m.   Judith wakes and immediately begins crying
            'Mummy coming.' Staff: 'Here we go again -
            do change your tune, Judith. Change it to
            Daddy for my sake.'

7.30   Sister coming around ward, children mostly
            talking and playing quietly on bed, except
            Judith - crying.

9.05   Judith put back in cot by cleaners immediately
            begins crying 'Mummy coming soon' again and
            screaming.

9.44	Judith standing up in cot crying as usual.
10.08	Staff goes to Judith and says to her cries: 'Of course she's coming' and does up the buttons on her dressing gown. At once her tune changes to 'Take it off me' but no one pays attention. She struggles with the dressing gown and after a couple of minutes has worked it off.
10.19	Dr J. comes to Judith and says 'Yes, she's coming' to J's cries; then to Staff: 'Put her in a cubicle.'
10.25	Sian walks down with the trolley (for traction). Judith lifted out to push trolley as well.
10.35	Judith comes back from C, picks up book, sits on chair and starts 'reading' to herself.
10.37	Mark is crying loudly. Judith wanders off down corridor. Nurse 12 catches her and takes her into a cubicle. Now saying, not crying, 'Mummy's coming now.' The nurse takes her to talk to Mary but she goes down corridor and plays with sliding door.
10.51	Judith is pushing the trolley around and talks to Nurse 6 sensibly - What a change.
11.00	Judith wanders round, pulls Mary's traction weights, she sits up and rearranges so weights rest on the rails.
12.56 p.m.	After dinner all in bed but Judith is crying as before.
1.01	Sister and Nurse 6 make bed B2. They won't pay attention to Judith.
2.27	Judith awake and crying: 'Mummy coming.'
2.42	Staff has Judith walking down corridor.
2.48	Judith's parents arrive.
3.21	Judith's parents have taken her out of the ward.
3.55	Judith walking with parents in corridor, visiting friends in cubicles.
4.23	Judith's mother and Sian's come to talk to Annette who tells them about her blood test. 'There's brave, you are,' they say.
5.20	Judith puts mother's poncho on, Nurse 6 says, 'There's lovely.' First words of praise for her?
6.31	Judith is back in cot, crying 'Mummy's coming.' Mother has gone.
6.45	Mother of Sian tries to interest Judith but she won't stop.
7.21	Judith is singing to herself.

Some further excerpts

From the third day

6.55 a.m.	Judith again: 'Mummy's coming now.'
7.01	Judith crying, 'Mummy coming. There we are.'
7.05	Nurses change Judith, whom they call 'misery'. (Mary praised for dry bed.) Red-haired Staff says, 'Oh Judith, change your tune. Can't you say, "Daddy's coming"?'
7.06	Student nurse tells Judith Mummy won't come if she hears her crying all the time.
11.02	Judith crying, Brian expresses his irritation: 'Mum's not coming. No good calling her if she's in the house. Funny girl. She gets on my nerves.' Wayne says: 'I'll smash her if she goes on screaming.'
2.35 p.m.	Two nurses walking and cuddling Sian. Teacher and receptionist at David's bed. Judith is still crying.

From the fifth day

8.01 p.m.	Judith cries off and on but no one pays attention. Why not? There are volunteers nearby talking to Susan and Diane.

From the sixth day

6.45 a.m.	Judith has started 'Mummy coming now.'
7.00	Brian and Elizabeth discuss Judith's crying. Anne says, 'Judith can't go home because she's bad (meaning ill, I think). The doctors will make her better.' Nurse asks Gerald what his teddy is called - 'Teddy.' 'That figures.' Asks Judith, 'Who's coming?' To other nurse: 'This child's like a parrot.'
7.20	Judith walking with Night Sister and student nurse, varies cry with 'Hello Mummy' and 'Oh, don't leave me here' and 'Here we are.' Put back into cot - gets more and more frantic, throwing things out of cot; screams when nurses are out of sight.
11.15	During consultant's round. Judith cries continuously, 'Mummy's coming now. I love her, she loves me, Mummy's coming.'
12.15	Judith still crying, 'Mummy's coming. I love her.'

On the seventh day, Judith was moved to a cubicle, where she remained for another six days.

Hawthorn (1974) found that in the wards she studied the category of time spent 'miserable and alone' correlated significantly and negatively with the quality of care given. The only positive reaction to the prolonged expression of unhappiness in this case was Judith's eventual removal to a cubicle, thus cutting her off from the opportunities for companionship and activity which sometimes distracted her during the absence of her parents. As the Staff Nurse said about Richard, 'When they're in a cubicle you can shut the door and get a bit of peace.'

Because of the organisation of nursing care in the ward, there was no one to alleviate her distress, and her admission came before the appointment of the playleader, who might have been able to help this 2½ year old. Her style of crying, the reiterated 'Mummy's coming soon', reflected the way in which passing nurses tended to react to children crying for their mothers - with the response 'Mummy's coming soon', perhaps three or four of them, one after the other - another instance of fragmented care.

The case studies (Hall, 1977) showed that children under 5 exhibited greater post-hospital disturbance than older children, and those with previous hospital experience were likely to be disturbed at the subsequent admission. Judith was such a child, having had several previous admissions and almost certain to have more, being hydrocephalic. She was in fact readmitted during the following month.

Douglas (1975), following up the 1946 cohort, presents evidence that one admission before the age of 5, lasting longer than a week, or several shorter ones, are associated with an increased risk of difficulties in adolescence, like poor reading ability and behavioural problems, both in school and out, including delinquency and job instability. It must be said, however, that those children would have been in hospital at a period when most hospitals were firmly wedded to the idea that visitors were undesirable for children and imposed severe restrictions or prohibitions in the interests of 'settling down'. Hopefully a study based on the 1970 cohort might present less disastrous results.

TASK ASSIGNMENT AND THE FRAGMENTATION OF CARE

Task assignment as a way of organising nursing care is particularly unsuitable for a children's ward. Etherington (1970): 'Each nurse feels she is doing her bit and literally she is; she attended to one part, her colleagues to another, but who attended to the whole patient?' Attention is routinely available around meal times and

toileting but is otherwise not easy to procure on the
child's initiative, since any nurse appearing in the ward
is probably doing something, something else from the child's
point of view.

The nurse's view of what is happening to any particular
child is necessarily fragmented and, while she is concentrating on a nursing task with one child, she tends to view the
others as children rather than patients, of whose activities
she is not fully aware. Consequently, situations can
develop that are distressing, clinically unhelpful, even
dangerous. Children come to rely upon their visitors and
each other for their needs, and this comes to be accepted
by staff, perhaps to an undesirable extent since these
helpers have been given little or no instruction in what
should be done. The child who is inarticulate or in-
competent, whether by reason of age, shyness, brain damage
or retardation, is at a disadvantage, and if this is
aggravated by a lack of visitors, the child may miss out
on all but basic care.

It is difficult to see just how these problems can be
overcome, although the first priority must be to keep young
children out of hospital as far as possible, by postponing
elective procedures, making use of day-care facilities
(Lawrie, 1964) and paediatric home-nursing schemes
(Robottom, 1969). Nevertheless, there will always be some
children whose episodes of acute illness require inpatient
treatment. The admission of mothers with their young
children has been recommended since the Platt Report
(Ministry of Health, 1959), but many hospitals (Hawthorn,
1974) feel their accommodation too inadequate to permit it
with any regularity and their staffs still find the presence
of the mothers difficult to accept or find them difficult
to integrate into the children's care, despite the evidence
from Kentucky and Indiana (James and Wheeler, 1969; Lerner
et al., 1972). Many mothers, on the other hand, are unconvinced of the necessity, or find that their other family
commitments make it virtually impossible for them to
accompany their children to hospital.

Within the ward, the presence of a nurse or other member
of the staff at all times might prevent the development
of episodes of aggression, if the observation of the
children was a principal call upon the nurses' attention
rather than a residual function. This supervision is
necessary at those periods of the day, early and late, when
there are normally relatively few members of staff on duty
and visiting is discouraged. The employment of more staff
would not, in itself, improve matters, without a change of
orientation, as the work of New et al. (1965) and Coser
(1963) suggests that staff-patient interaction is not

necessarily a function of the availability of staff, and
they are supported by Stockwell (1972) and Dodd (1973).
Increased numbers of staff would not help to reduce the
number of people dealing with each child or the fragmentation of care unless the organisation of work in the ward
were given a different orientation.

IMPROVING PATIENT CARE

Patient assignment (Hales-Tooke, 1973), team nursing
(Etherington, 1970) and primary nursing (Bakke, 1974;
Marram et al., 1974) have all been argued as ways to
improve the quality of patient care. The first - patient
assignment - is the most obviously suitable for child
patients, since each would then have an 'own' nurse, who
would have a less fragmented view of the child and the needs
of that child, and to whom the child could more easily turn
for help and reassurance, without always finding that the
nurse was doing 'something else'. The nurse's continuing
responsibility would be to her patient or patients, rather
than to a series of tasks, each of which is to be completed
for a batch of children. The demands of the existing shift
system and the staffing of children's wards principally by
students in training (mainly for the General Register), make
the system difficult to administer but not, in the opinion
of ward Sisters who use it, impossible. If senior staff are
convinced of the necessity, it can be done. A parallel
can be drawn with mothering-in, a policy most consistently
followed where the conviction is strongest rather than the
facilities most lavish, as has been shown, for example, at
Amersham and the Brook Hospital (MacCarthy et al., 1962;
also McElnea, 1971, reporting on Great Ormond Street).
It may be that the difficulties imposed by shift working
can be partially overcome by incorporating elements from
team nursing and primary nursing, by creating an across-
shift team. Another North American system of working is a
reorganisation of working hours into what might be called a
long-day/short-week pattern. A 10-12 hour day is worked for
a 'week' of perhaps four days followed by a break of roughly
the same length (De Marsh and McLellan, 1971; Staples and
Curtis, 1975). A nurse assigned to a newly admitted child
on her first day of duty would be able to see more than half
the child patients in an acute general hospital through their
stay and be present throughout the normal waking day.
Non-nursing staff can make a great contribution to the
children's welfare: a 'ward granny' (Jolly, 1974) would have
been of great assistance to a child like Judith, but they
are unlikely to be employed on a wide scale. Play and

education staff are invaluable for the older and longer-stay children, not only for the expertise they can provide but because they are child-orientated and are, unlike nurses in training, long-term workers in the ward (Hales-Tooke, 1973; Noble, 1967; Petrillo and Sanger, 1972; Plank, 1964). However, financial considerations make it unlikely that many hospitals will be able to extend provision to cover the ends of the day or the weekends (DHSS, 1976a).

While it must be said that the evidence presented comes from one ward in one hospital, it is a typical ward in a typical hospital. It may be that its standards were low compared with those of the very best hospitals but it would be unrealistic to assume that it was unique. Many hospitals, particularly teaching hospitals, are able to provide the highest quality of care, welcoming mothers and able to give day-long care by play personnel, but it must be remembered that most children (and adults) are admitted to general hospitals that cannot aspire to such standards: in 1972, of all admissions 85 per cent were to non-teaching hospitals (DHSS and OPCS, 1974).

To conclude, although it is possible to reduce the number of inpatient admissions among children, it seems likely that for most of those whose admission is inevitable, care will remain principally in the hands of the nursing staff for the foreseeable future. In order to lessen distress within hospital, to cut down the number of clinically unhelpful events and reduce undesirable behavioural sequelae, both short and long term, it will be necessary to change the orientation and the organisation of the work within the ward, so that it will provide a more satisfactory response to the needs of the child patient.

CHAPTER SIX

Status and Career

A sociological approach to the study of child patients

Roisin Pill

INTRODUCTION

'Life-chance' is one of the most fundamental concepts in
sociology. From the moment of its birth into a particular
family, every child may be regarded as having particular
avenues open to it, while, conversely, others will be closed.
Colour, sex, caste are thus all life-chances, and their
implications will vary from society to society. Tradition-
ally, sociologists have explored the significance of
membership of social groups based on cultural, ethnic or
socio-economic criteria for the child's career in education,
his eventual occupational attainment, choice of marriage
partner, and life-style.

Knowledge of an individual's social position also
improves prediction of his life-chances in the most literal
sense because of the well-known correlations between social
class, for example, and mortality and morbidity rates.
Much of the work of medical sociologists has been devoted
to the description of such ethnic and class variations, and
efforts to elucidate the underlying factors have often
concentrated on attempts to explore the relationships
between attitudes towards illness and health-care facilities
and utilisation of the services (Koos, 1954; Anderson and
Andersen, 1972). The general perspective underlying this
work stresses that patterns of illness behaviour (1) are
the product of social and cultural conditioning.

In the following pages it is argued that health itself
can be regarded as a life-chance which has potentially as
much relevance for socialisation as membership of an ethnic
or socio-economic group. Children who are ascribed different
health statuses are likely to follow quite different educational and occupational careers and, of course, to have
different patterns of relationship with the health services.
This is not to deny the importance of the ethnic and

socio-economic variables, but is to make a case for
considering the interrelationship of these factors with
health. Such a perspective has implications for the
analysis of the behaviour of the child and his family,
and is relevant to questions of social policy and the
efficacy of the welfare state in providing health and
social services according to need.

THE CONCEPT OF HEALTH STATUS

The sociological perspective has treated health as a norm
and, following Parsons' (1958) definition, we can define
health as 'the state of optimum capacity of an individual
for the effective performance of the roles and tasks for
which he has been socialised. It is thus defined with
reference to the individual's participation in the social
system.' Obviously no one has perfect health and not
everyone is defined as ill, so there must be a range of
less than perfect health which is defined as normal. It
is here that social definitions become crucial.

Over the life-cycle, criteria for 'normal health' will
change, and within social and cultural groups different
expectations will hold about criteria for someone to be
called 'ill'. As noted, there is a large literature on
the negotiation process that takes place between the
individual and significant others (Freidson, 1961;
Knutson, 1965; Roth, 1963). During the life-cycle various
symptoms and signs will be experienced, interpreted, and
a course of action decided upon that may bring the
individual into contact with a doctor or other health agent.
Thus most of the population have a 'normal' health status,
follow a pattern of contact with health agencies that is
'normal' for their particular social grouping, and their
health allows them to achieve the roles that again are
'normal' for their position in society. (In the case of
children, of course, it is the parents' perceptions and
subsequent actions that are particularly relevant.)

This picture is altered if the individual is impaired
in some way either from birth or as the result of an illness
or trauma. However, impairment will not be socially
relevant unless those closest to the individual interpret
the disability as materially affecting the capacity to
assume appropriate roles either now or in the future (2).
Hitherto the concept of negotiation and the process of
designating someone as 'ill' have usually been employed for
a particular illness episode; but the same process also
takes place on a much larger scale in considering the
individual's overall fitness for the roles open to her/him.

From the time of birth the individual has certain physical
characteristics, colour, sex, the presence or absence of
disability, which provide the material for a process of
labelling to begin which will bring certain consequences
in its wake.

NEGOTIATING HEALTH STATUS

Certain children will have such a degree of impairment that
their parents and professionals may agree that they will
never be able to achieve social competence, that is, perform
in valued social roles. At the other end of the continuum
the majority of children will not exhibit any gross
physical or mental defects and will be regarded as 'normal'
although, as time passes, such a definition may have to be
re-negotiated if evidence to the contrary presents itself.
Within these extremes there is obviously the possibility
that the process of labelling may take different forms and
it is these that we will now examine.
There are two sets of people crucially involved in
negotiating about the child's health status - the parents
of the child and the doctors and other professionals.
It is usually considered desirable, from the point of view
of the wider society, that a consensus is arrived at,
between both sides, on the extent of disability and the
probable outcome in order that the child may be channelled
into the appropriate treatment programme or facilities,
where they exist. The sooner this occurs the better it
is deemed to be for the child.
Yet it is abundantly clear from research that a speedy
consensus may be the exception rather than the rule. Even
in cases where the parents accept the doctors' diagnosis
they may not be prepared to accept the implications as
conveyed by the doctor as representative of the community.
Advice to put the child in an institution, and statements
that the child will never be able to attend an ordinary
school, may well be rejected. Cases where the child is
not obviously disabled may also be difficult to accept.
At the other extreme doctors have also been criticised
for reluctance to commit themselves to predictions about
a child's potential. Davis (1963), for example, has
described how doctors structure their interaction with
the parents of polio victims, apparently hoping that the
truth about their child's condition and its consequences
will gradually dawn on them. On the other hand parents
may find difficulty in convincing their doctor that something is indeed wrong with their child. Both Hewett (1970)
and Burton (1975) report the frustration felt by mothers

when they were convinced that their child was not developing properly but were unable to obtain confirmation of their suspicions. In some cases this went on for years before a diagnosis was made; that is, a label was attached to the child, carrying prognostic implications of varying degrees of clarity and uncertainty.

There is some evidence of the relevance of social class to the labelling process. For example, in her study of children with cystic fibrosis Burton found a positive relationship between parental social class and the speed of the child's diagnosis. She attributes this to the greater intelligence, articulation and determination of parents in the professional and managerial classes (Social Classes I and II), who are less likely to be deflected by medical scepticism. The similarity in background between doctors and parents aids communication and such parents are more likely to obtain confirmation of their suspicions from textbooks and paediatric manuals, thus providing ammunition when pressing for the child's needs to be taken seriously.

So far the focus has been on variables affecting the *process* of labelling and it is argued that (a) the time at which a medical diagnosis is given and (b) the extent of a consensus between parents and professionals concerning the implications of the diagnosis are theoretically of great relevance to a child's subsequent career. Turning from the process to a consideration of the *content* of the label, we focus not on the clinical terminology but on the implications of a particular diagnosis in the assessment of a child's health status. The two relevant variables appear to be the severity of the impairment and the prognosis.

THE OPERATIONAL DEFINITION OF HEALTH STATUS

The operational problem of measuring impairment has generally been tackled in the context of assessing the amount and type of help that might be needed, usually concentrating on the extent to which the disability limits activities essential to daily living (Bennet et al., 1970; Katz et al., 1958). Attempts to measure functional impairment in children pose particular problems because of developmental and also cultural differences but, never-theless, it seems reasonable to set upper age limits by which most children are expected to cope with certain basic living activities themselves (Hewett, 1970). Five years of age, the time of starting school, is an obvious watershed since mothers will not be on hand to assist with feeding, toilet and dressing. Davis (1963) used a combination of degrees of self-care and mobility in his study of child polio victims, while Hewett also included communication difficulties in her study of spastics.

Bennett and associates concluded that detailed questioning about the level of daily performances is the most reliable method of identifying and measuring disability and, in the case of children, this approach can be defended on the grounds that it is the mother's description of what the disability means to her in practical terms that is relevant. Her reports are likely to be an accurate reflection of what the child is encouraged and allowed to do for himself, and thus to be a valid index of the degree of functional impairment.

The prognosis is the forecast of the outcome of the disease or the eventual extent of the impairment. For the purposes of the following analysis it has been decided to adopt Freidson's (1965) classification of imputed prognoses: curable, improvable but not curable, incurable and unimprovable. The significance of each of these for the child's future will obviously depend on the previous variable - extent of impairment. A child could well be born with a defect that could be classified as incurable and unimprovable but the defect might range from a slight deformation of an ear to gross physical and mental handicap. Table 6.1 sets out the logical possibilities arising from combinations of the two variables and it will be assumed, for the sake of ease of presentation, that this is the situation at birth. (3)

TABLE 6.1   Impairment and prognosis

Prognosis	Severity of impairment		
	Severe	Moderate	Slight/nil
Curable	A	B	C
Improvable	D	E	F
Incurable and unimprovable	G	H	I

Taking the view that health status is defined by assessing the individual's capacities for present or future role performance, the categories can be combined into three types of health status. Parents and professionals alike will adopt some model of the socially competent adult against which to measure individual children. In the broadest terms, social competence may be defined, following Inkeles (1966), as the ability to work at gainful and reasonably remunerative employment, to manage one's own affairs, to achieve some significant and effective participation in community and political life and to establish and maintain a reasonably stable home and family life. The parents of 'normal' children (C, F and I) have every reason to hope that their offspring will attain these valued social roles, whereas the parents of the most severly impaired, for whom little if anything can be done (D, G and H), will have every reason to doubt that. In between these extremes there are the children who are impaired now to the extent that the pattern of their lives is materially affected but who, on the other hand, can look forward to being as normal as their fellows in time. At any rate, treatment may ensure that they have the potential for achieving some degree of independence by looking after and supporting themselves financially.

The argument put forward here is that a health status is negotiated for the child as the result of interaction between the child's family and the professionals. This is based on estimates of present and particularly future capacity to achieve independence and valued adult roles, and rests largely on perception of the severity of impairment and prognosis. (Acute illness episodes common to all children are ignored in assigning health status and only become relevant if they result in a degree of impairment sufficiently severe to necessitate a re-negotiation of health status.) The process of negotiation itself and the status ascribed may crucially affect the child's socialisation and the institutions and agencies with which the child comes into contact. Thus, health status influences not only the way in which the child is handled but the range and type of experiences to which the child is exposed. This point will be developed later in the analysis of reaction to hospital, both in the ward and on the return home.

TREATMENT CAREER

One of the most obvious differences in the type of experience to which children of different health status are likely to be exposed is the pattern of contact with health professionals and agencies. Such patterns are referred to in this chapter as 'treatment careers'. The concept of 'career' was originally developed by sociologists in studies of occupations and referred to the sequence of movements from one position to another in an occupational system made by any individual who worked in that system (Hughes, 1958; Hall, 1948). It also includes

the notion of 'career contingency', that is those factors
on which mobility from one position to another depends.
Contingencies may include objective facts of social
structure and changes in the perspectives, motivations
and desires of the individual and may thus be used to
distinguish several varieties of career outcome (Becker,
1963).

The suggestion is that standardised sequences of contact
with health agencies are discernible for various categories
of children and that certain factors will lead to particular
children receiving one treatment sequence rather than
another. However, it is important to realise that although
there will obviously be gross differences between children
of differing health status, there is great variation in
treatment careers within the same health-status category,
and even within the same diagnostic category.

This point is illustrated by taking hospital admission
as an example of a treatment provision and considering
some of the possible sequences of contact for children of
different health status.

(a) The 'normal' children

These are children whose state of health has not constrained them in any way. They suffer the usual childish
ailments and mishaps but recover completely. Any contact
they have with hospital is likely to be of a routine
nature - for example, for observation or a minor operation -
and short in duration. Where they have been admitted more
than once it is likely that it will be for quite different
reasons. There is some evidence that, in cases where
discretion can be exercised over admission, there is a
tendency to admit more children from Social Classes IV and V.
The parents of higher socio-economic status seem to be
regarded as more capable of looking after the child
properly at home, both in the material and medical senses.

(b) The moderately impaired children

These are children who may have been disabled from birth
or who have become disabled as the result of accident or
illness. It is possible that they may be permanently in
hospital if family circumstances are unfavourable, but it
is more likely that they will be used to a pattern of a
number of admissions during childhood. Some children with
chronic conditions such as diabetes or asthma may have to
enter hospital in an acute episode, while others may have

to undergo corrective surgery. In the latter case, there
is scope for considerable variation in medical practice
as to whether children are treated mainly at a clinic or
in a hospital and, if admitted, whether they are kept in
hospital for a long period or sent home sooner and recalled
for regular check-ups (Harrisson, 1974; Clough, 1975).

(c) The severely impaired children

Again these children may be impaired from birth or may
have become impaired later in childhood. They may have
been hospitalised from the beginning or may have been
cared for almost entirely at home if there was little that
medical intervention could do. Frequent admissions may
be for corrective surgery or simply to give relief to a
family that increasingly finds the care of such a severely
handicapped child too great a burden. One of the admissions
may eventually be protracted and the child may stay in
hospital indefinitely. This is more likely to happen
as the child grows older and the differences between the
child and its peers become more marked and the implications
of the child's state are borne in on the family.
      As sociologists we are interested in explaining why
some children follow one sequence of movements between the
social networks comprised in the terms 'hospital' and
'home' and some follow another. It is apparent that some
of the variation is due to differences in medical practice:
one consultant may routinely treat his patients at outpatient
clinics and admit only when he feels the time is right for
surgical intervention, while another will bring the child
in for treatment on every occasion. However, there is
considerable evidence to suggest the relevance of social
and psychological variables and again we return to the
concept of the negotiation process between the parents
and the health professionals.

THE PARENTS' ROLE

It is impossible to ignore the role of the parents in every
aspect of the child's treatment career. Usually it is they
who originally present the child for medical scrutiny and
thus initiate the first step towards treatment. Their
choice of a doctor may radically affect the pattern of
treatment offered to them (Clough, 1975) and the nature
of the relationship they form with the doctor may also
affect its course. The doctor's perceptions of the understanding and competence of the parents will sometimes

influence the decision to admit in the first place and
may also affect the time of discharge. Parents from
different social and ethnic backgrounds may well experience
problems in handling relations with their child's doctor
and it is here, as noted earlier, that middle-class parents,
who are also more likely to possess relevant interpersonal
skills, will have an advantage.

Voysey (1975) goes so far as to argue that acquisition
of a special competence in managing such encounters is
likely to be one of the consequences of having a child
whose health status is not normal. Such parents can
expect to have a continuing relationship with health-care
services and other agencies, and learn appropriate
strategies of 'impression management' to obtain what they
want from professionals.

Obviously the extent to which parents consciously attempt
to control the outcome of their encounters with health professionals, and thus affect the treatment pattern, will
vary according to their knowledge of alternatives, the
value they place on a particular type of treatment or
treatment setting, and the implications they foresee for the
child and the rest of the family. Whether or not impression
management is deliberately employed, the doctor will
certainly form an impresssion of the parents, which may
well affect decisions as to the mode and setting for
treatment. Health status is important in so far as both
sides' perceptions of it and its implications provide a
framework for the negotiation that takes place at a
particular time.

THE CAREER PERSPECTIVE

The career concept is potentially useful since it provides
a way of analysing change and the impact of the passage
of time. One might view a person's whole life as a bundle
of interlocking careers, each one following its own
particular timetable (Roth, 1963). Thus interruption or
gross distortion in one area will naturally affect the others.

Children's treatment careers may radically affect
their educational and social and developmental careers.
Moreover, there will be implications for other members of
the family because, in so far as the individual career
timetables of family members are expected to form a
reasonably well-integrated whole, one which is discrepant
with the others and does not develop and progress in the
normal way poses a conflict for the members which needs
resolution. A great deal of the literature is concerned
precisely with this topic - how parents deal with the

problem of a disabled child - but inevitably the majority
is surveys of a cross-section of ages (Hewett, 1970;   Burton,
1975;   Davis, 1963).   Changes in the parents' attitudes
and behaviour over time have to be studied retrospectively
with all the disadvantages of this technique.   There are
no longitudinal studies which explore the process of how
the parents structure their situation over time.   Aspects
of their lives may be substantially influenced by the fact
that their child is not following a 'normal' health career.
For example, the mother may have planned to go back to
work as soon as the children were old enough, or the parents
may decide against a move to another area which would take
them away from known and respected medical advisors and
the help of family and friends.

MORAL CAREERS AND TREATMENT CAREERS

Thus the career concept has both a subjective and an
objective component.   On the one hand it focuses our
attention on the standardised sequences of moves from one
network of relationships to another, and this is the aspect
stressed above in the discussion of treatment career.
Such an approach leads one to ask questions as to why a
particular sequence is followed rather than another, and
possibly to investigate the consequences of this for
individuals and those involved with them.   On the other
hand certain sociologists, notably Goffman (1961), have
been more interested in the 'moral career' of the individual,
that is, the standard sequence of changes in the way given
social categories perceive themselves and others (in the
case of mental patients).   Goffman argued that one could
examine moral experiences, that is, happenings which
marked a turning point in the way the individual viewed
the world and overt stands and strategies employed, and
thus obtain a relatively objective tracing of relatively
subjective matters.
    The interrelationship between children's moral careers
in this sense and their treatment careers offers an exciting
field for investigation but little has been done in this
area, although Clough (1975 and chapter 3 above) has shown
how important it is for an adequate understanding of the
child's reactions to hospital to probe the meanings that
the child attaches to home, parents, other patients, and so
on.   The concept of moral career would also seem potentially
fruitful in the analysis of parental perceptions over time.
I have argued that health status is ascribed as the result
of negotiations between parents and professionals and that
subsequently treatment career is affected by such negotiations.

The 'meaning' of children's health status to their parents will change over time: children will inevitably alter as a result of their experiences, and the parents' perceptions of them and their definition of the situation will change, thus influencing the next stage of the treatment career.

Hitherto medical sociologists have tended to restrict career to the concept of 'patient career', referring generally to a simple illness episode, and they have focused on thé factors underlying varying patterns of illness behaviour. It is suggested here that the concepts of health status and treatment career have potential for the analysis of the behaviour of child patients and their families and are capable of much wider application. The rest of the chapter attempts to substantiate this claim by showing how career perspective can be used (a) to analyse the situation of a particular category of child patient, namely long-stay children, and (b) to interpret the reactions, in the ward and post-hospital, of a sample of children in an orthopaedic hospital.

THE LONG-STAY CHILD

Disadvantages of hospital stay

It is apparent that the category of long-stay children is linked in the minds of many health professionals and administrators with the word 'problem'. Some recognise that a long period in hospital, in the words of the Platt Report (Ministry of Health, 1959), creates particular problems for the child because of prolonged separation from home and parents and because of the need for the child to become fully adjusted to the life of the hospital. Studies by Oswin (1971) and King, Raynes and Tizard (1971) have demonstrated that the quality of life experienced by children in hospital compares unfavourably with that experienced by children of similar health status in other forms of residential long-term care. Moreover, they were able to relate the poor quality of care directly to features of the hospital organisation and staff training, and such findings must necessarily raise the whole question of the suitability of in-hospital treatment for children, particularly for long periods. Where hospital treatment is unavoidable, doctors, nurses and administrators will have to give thought to altering the traditional ward patterns of care so that they do not violate the practices followed in the best child-care establishments.

Reason for long stay

Under these circumstances it becomes especially important
that no one is admitted for long periods unless it is
strictly medically necessary. There is evidence that the
Department of Health and Social Security is concerned about
the proportion of long-stay child patients in for other
reasons (4) since, apart from considerations of a child's
welfare, such admissions also represent a misuse of hospital
resources. Three main reasons have been recognised as
contributing to the length of a child's stay: first,
variation in medical practice, which sometimes leads to
considerable differences in length of hospital treatment
second, the need for education which might not have been
possible outside hospital; and third, social reasons,
that is, all the other factors to do with the child's
background and family circumstances. It is difficult to
escape the conclusion that this last reason is used as a
residual category for all that cannot be explained in any
other way.

Numbers of long-stay children

In an attempt to determine the size of the problem, the
Department of Health and Social Security carried out a
survey in 1967 of children in non-psychiatric wards in
NHS hospitals. The definition adopted for 'long stay' was
'children under the age of 15 who have been or are likely
to be in a hospital as in-patients for a period of at least
four months, absences of short holiday periods being
ignored' (DHSS, mimeo, 1970). The number of children that
fell into this category was 1,561, or roughly 8 per cent
of the total child in-patient population (5). The most
numerous groups, by main diagnosis, were 181 spina bifida
cases (12.4 per cent of the total), 180 children with
perthes disease (12.3 per cent), 164 with musculo-skeletal
diseases (11.2 per cent), 119 with asthma (8.1 per cent)
and 117 suffering from cerebral palsy (8.0 per cent).

DEFINITIONAL DIFFICULTIES

The first point to make is that the definition adopted by
the DHSS is an administrative one and, as such, is of little
use for research purposes. Any definition of a particular
population using length of stay as the sole measure is bound
to produce a very heterogeneous group. First, it will
include all those conditions for which the prescribed

length of stay is the average time spent in hospital and, second, it will include those staying longer than the norm for their particular condition for some reason, which may be medical but which may also be due to social and psychological factors.   It is likely, therefore, that the longer the period taken as the definition of 'long stay', the fewer the number of patients who will fall into the first group and the greater the number that will fall into the second, especially since the average time in hospital for all children is between nine and ten days. (6)

According to the DHSS definition long-stay child patients are comparatively few in number, scattered and very heterogeneous with regard to diagnosis and prognosis.   But these children can represent only a small proportion of their diagnostic grouping in the hospital population and an even smaller percentage of the total population of physically handicapped children, which has been estimated as being one-twelfth of the total child population (Packman and Power, 1968).   Thus, to use the terminology employed in this chapter, the administrative definition of 'long stay' will produce a category of children of very different health status and treatment career, while many children with directly comparable status and treatment career will not fall into this category.   The argument is that the simple dichotomy, 'short stay' versus 'long stay', is essentially a static, hospital-oriented frame of reference and of little use in (a) predicting which children are at risk of becoming long stay in the DHSS sense and (b) aiding analysis of the problems faced by their families.

SOCIAL IMPLICATIONS OF LONG STAY

Children in hospital for 4 months or more may have had a normal health status up until that time and the prognosis for this episode may be good or may imply that a new status will have to be negotiated.   All parents may experience problems of re-adjustment when a child has been away for a time, and this will be compounded when the child returns with a residue of handicap.   Davis (1963) has described graphically the situation facing the families of polio victims and the strategies they employed: he found that, where there had been considerable impairment, re-adjustment became much more difficult, prolonged and pervasive.

Many of the long-stay children will not have normal health status and again the prognosis may be more or less hopeful.   Impairment and its consequences is something that the parents may well have had to cope with since the birth of the child, and long periods in hospital may be just one of a host of related problems - for example, special schooling, frequent visits to the clinic, special diets, shoes and equipment (McMichael, 1971). The children may well have been in hospital on previous occasions, even if they were not long-stay patients, in the administrative sense, each time.

Because of the period of time involved, visiting can impose quite severe strains on the financial and emotional resources of all the families of long-stay children. In a survey conducted by the Welsh Hospital Board (Stacey and Earthrowl, 1973) it was found that 42 per cent of long-stay child patients, compared with 16 per cent of the main survey respondents, reported that getting transport to hospital presented a problem; 46 per cent compared with 27 per cent reported that cost of transport was a difficult problem; 30 per cent compared with 21 per cent had difficulties in arranging for other children to be minded. Nevertheless, in the majority of cases, the family may expect to have the child home in a matter of months rather than years. Visiting raises particular problems with the relatively small number of severely impaired children who, in the foreseeable future, will always need care and may remain in hospital for years. The parents have to decide what kind of relationship to maintain with their child, recognising that in some cases the child's life expectancy is severely limited while others may have no social future in the sense that they will not be able to attain and perform valued social roles. Visiting every weekend for an indefinite period represents a tremendous commitment of time and resources by the family. If parents are no longer responsible for the care of their child and if the child is incapable of remembering or recognising them, the basis for any relationship becomes extremely tenuous. Infrequency of visiting may reflect disinterest but may also arise because visiting is found to be too painful.

LONG-STAY CHILDREN IN WELSH HOSPITALS

The following data from the survey of children in hospital in Wales offer an opportunity to explore and illustrate some of these propositions. In January 1972, enquiry of all the relevant hospitals showed that there were 261 children who were long stay. The majority was mentally handicapped, only 29 being in non-psychiatric hospitals, and interviews with the parents of 26 of these were completed. Table 6.2 sets out the diagnosis, together with variables discussed earlier as being relevant to health status.

TABLE 6.2   Long-stay children: some health-status variables

No.	Diagnosis	Time of labelling	Degree of impairment before admission	Prognosis
5	Multiply handicapped	Birth	Severe	Incurable/ unimprovable
2	Physical handicap only	Birth	Severe	Improvable?
1	CDH	2 years	Moderate	Curable
1	CDH	Birth	Moderate	Curable
1	Perthes disease	2 years	Slight	Curable
6	Asthma	Early childhood	Variable	Improvable/ controllable
8	TB	Recent	Nil	Curable
2	Accidents	Recent	Nil	?

Out of this sample of 26 children the majority appeared to be in hospital for primarily medical reasons. This was undoubtedly the case for the TB and trauma cases and for 5 of the asthma patients (57 per cent of the total). There were only three cases (11 per cent) in which there was unambiguous evidence that had it not been for the family situation the child would have returned home. The mother of a 3-year-old boy suffering from asthma was unable to say when she would take him home, since her husband had left her and she had to find accommodation for herself and two younger children. Another physically handicapped boy of 5 had been in hospital for more than two years. He was the youngest of four children and his mother was separated from her husband and living on social security. She had gone to see the specialist and asked if the child could be admitted for a while as she did not feel fit enough to look after him. She claimed to have domestic troubles, to be suffering from nerves and to be about to undergo an operation. The other children had been taken into care. At the time of the interview they were living with her and she told the interviewer that she could have the hospitalised child home at anytime but she hadn't room at the moment and had 'lost her nerve'.

In both these cases the hospital was really being used for care not cure, and although the consultants involved may have felt that they were helping the situation this is open to debate. The third case was a child with perthes

disease, who had been kept in because of his inability to
stop breaking his plaster. His mother had two other
children and found him difficult to handle; apparently it
was her failure to cope with looking after the plaster and
controlling the child which led to his retention.

HOSPITAL OR HOME?

When we examine the position of the most severely impaired
children, the picture is more complicated because there is
no doubt that these children make heavy demands on nursing
care and could therefore be classified as needing
hospitalisation. Yet it is clear that there are children
who are equally handicapped being looked after at home.
In this little group there is no evidence that they have
been admitted for educational reasons or for the type of
social reason described above, that is, single-parent
families, lack of money and accommodation. One might have
expected that the families of the children in hospital
would be more disadvantaged materially and would have
family structures different from those that kept their
children at home, but this does not appear necessarily to
be the case. In looking for differences in the family
background of severely subnormal hospitalised and non-
hospitalised children, Hewett (1972) found that there were
no significant variations for the two samples in family
size or the proportion of single-parent families. The
most significant factors in her study were the greater
proportions of mothers in the hospital sample who reported
their husbands as being non-supportive, either psycho-
logically or practically, and who expressed concern about
the adverse effect the handicapped child was having on their
marriage and on siblings.
     This appears to lend support to the argument put forward
earlier in the chapter that it is the parents' perception
that is important: their perception of the impact that the
child is having on their lives, the implications for their
own timetables now and in the future, after the decision
to put the child in hospital, or, alternatively, not to
press for discharge. In this context, reports of marital
stress and of disturbance among the other children may be
seen as the appropriate reasons to put forward in dealing
with doctors and others. This is not to deny the
importance of these factors, but rather to emphasise the
interaction process and the impression management involved.
All but one of the most severely impaired were not expected
to come home in the foreseeable future, so the parents had
made a decision, consciously or by default, that the child
should receive institutional care.

To sum up, there is evidence that children are at risk
of becoming long-stay patients through the very factors which
may lead to admission in the first place. If the family
has no more than a single parent, or the father is out-of-
work, unskilled or poorly educated, the family may well
have other health, accommodation and financial problems.
The parent(s) will not be in such a strong position to
deal with professionals as higher-status families will and,
in cases where they may want to have their child home
their impression-management techniques may not succeed
with staff, who often categorise such homes as 'unsuitable'
and the adults as incapable of giving proper care. Once
admitted such children run the risk of links with home becoming attenuated over time, since visiting problems are
likely to impose considerable financial burdens on families
with limited means and to impose unacceptable emotional
burdens on parents who do not wish their child to return.
The most severely impaired children, who are always going
to need considerable care, are also at risk of becoming
long stay regardless of their health status or the
resources available to their families. As we have seen,
the exact stage at which this occurs in the child's
treatment career will depend on the outcome of negotiations
by parents and professionals about the future, and upon
the parents' assessment and valuation of the impact of the
child's health status on the rest of the family.

THE REACTIONS OF CHILDREN DURING AND AFTER HOSPITALISATION:
EXAMPLES FROM AN ORTHOPAEDIC WARD

Aim of study

In our study of children on an orthopaedic ward we started
from the position that children of differing health status,
and therefore very probably different treatment careers,
would vary in their behaviour on the ward and in the extent
of post-hospital disturbance as measured by behavioural
ratings completed by the mother and, where applicable, the
teacher. The theoretical basis for this hypothesis
stemmed from the original research in which one of the
major propositions was that the child's behaviour in
hospital would be the combined result of the person he
had become before entry and the impact upon him of the
social system encountered in the hospital (Stacey et al.
1970). It was recognised that the child was being reared
in a social network comprising the several systems or sub-
systems of family, kin and neighbourhood and that each
potentially could affect the expectations of behaviour
acquired.

The original studies found relationships between children's reactions in the ward setting and certain aspects of family structure and child-rearing practice: those children reared in households consisting of some form of the extended family were more likely to exhibit atypical reactions and there was some suggestion that the parents of children who displayed normal reactions were more authoritarian than than those whose children were atypical. These tentative findings direct our attention to the characteristics of socialisation settings and the way in which they facilitate or inhibit the individual's capacity to adapt or adjust to new settings.

Interpersonal competence

It was hypothesised in the first study that the child entered hospital with sets of expectations which might or might not be appropriate for the new roles he or she would be called upon to play; thus we had implicitly assumed that the *content* of the expectations was the most relevant factor.   However, our perspective would now emphasise the extent of mastery of interpersonal skills, what Goslin has called 'socialisation for socialisation' (Goslin, 1969). It is argued that an important part of the socialisation process is the acquisition of certain skills that will facilitate subsequent role-learning and performance. Goslin points out that verbal skills, ability to perceive oneself as others perceive one and ability to differentiate between real and ideal role-expectations are likely to be necessary for role-learning, and that obvious differences between individuals' cognitive and verbal status will exist as a function of age, prior training and experience.
    Such interpersonal skills can only be developed through interaction.   Therefore, children who differ in the range and type of previous interaction experience might be expected to show different levels of interpersonal competence when faced with a new situation.   Interpersonal competence here means the ability to shape the responses of others (Foote and Cottrell, 1955; Weinstein, 1969). Thus the skills needed are those which enable people to get others to think, feel, or do what they want them to. Two crucial skills are, first, the ability to predict correctly the impact that various lines of action will have on another's definition of the situation, that is, the ability to take the role of the other accurately and, secondly, the ability to display a repertoire of effective tactics. (7)
    It may be assumed that a child who is exposed to a

breadth and variety of social relationships is likely to
develop a greater accuracy in role-taking; first, because
one of the best ways to improve the capacity to take a
given role is to have played it oneself, and second, the
greater the variety of social situations encountered the
more the firsthand acquaintance with the exigencies of role
behaviour in such situations. The corollary of this
proposition is that those whose life chances for one reason
or another restrict the experiences that facilitate role-
taking accuracy and will be less successful in developing
interpersonal skills.

There is certainly evidence that children whose health
status differs from the normal have a more restricted range
of interaction experiences. Physically handicapped
children experience such restrictions either because parents
limit the opportunities available or because functional
restrictions inhibit the formation of voluntary relationships. It seems that children quickly learn the cultural
values pertaining to physical disability and that these
prejudices find behavioural expression (Richardson et al.,
1961). Despite what they are taught, normal children do
not easily accept disabled children (Centers and Centers,
1963). Data from other studies suggest that the kind of
people who generally make friends with a disabled child are
those who are less successful in social relations themselves,
those who hold atypical values, those for whom disability
cues have low perceptual salience or those who like others
to be dependent on them (Richardson, 1969). Our own data
from the orthopaedic ward, using interviews with the mother,
clearly showed that the more severly impaired the child,
the more likely he or she was to receive special treatment,
particularly in matters of discipline, and the more likely
to be reported as being 'very shy' with strange adults and
the less likely to have contact with other children.

Thus handicapped children whose health status is
abnormal may experience a more restricted range of social
settings than their normal peers and the quality of their
interaction may also differ which, one may hypothesise,
would lead to problems in the development of role-taking
skills. Furthermore such children are often deprived of
the normal interaction with peers, which Weinstein (1969)
would argue is essential for the acquisition of a suitable
range of tactics. Children observe and then can attempt to
control outcomes in their relations with other children.
Notions of reciprocity among equals and bargaining
situations within the peer group can sensitise the child
to the cues which indicate the outcome values held by the
others and the kind of resources the child can use to
trade for what he or she wants.

Interpersonal skills in the ward

Communication skills assume vital importance in a ward
situation, particularly where a majority of the children
is bedfast all the time.   Tactics for attracting attention
are therefore important.   The prime one used by the younger
children was simply to cry.   However, its success varied
according to the definition placed on it by the nursing
staff: if it was evaluated as a cry of pain it received
prompt attention, but if it was interpreted as a cry for
parents it might be ignored, particularly if previous
attention had not resulted in stopping distress.   Similarly,
the older children might call out to the nurse, who had
her own categories for assessing the priorities for action.
Children judged to be in pain, especially after treatment
procedures, were attended first.   It was clear that the
nurses' definitions changed over time, since a child who
received a lot of sympathy and attention over the first
few days might find that constant demands would not be met
with the same quick response later.   Then the nurses
attempted to re-define the child's role by stressing the
need for self-control and using notions about the levels
of stoicism appropriate for particular age and sex
characteristics: 'Come on now, you're a big girl.'
     Among the youngest children, therefore, there was little
observable difference between the health-status categories
in the extent of interaction they had with nurses and peers
which could reasonably be attributed to degrees of social
skills.   Age is a vital factor since cognitive development
is intimately linked with language learning, the ability
to role-play and the development of empathy.   For the
youngest children interaction with nurses was largely
governed by the children's dependency status;   there was
little they could do to control what happened to them and
the tactics at their disposal were generally rudimentary.
Interaction with older children was very limited because
of lack of communication skills, and the immobility of the
majority.
     Once children can talk, however, differences among the
health-status categories do begin to emerge and these are
now described in greater detail.

THE ORTHOPAEDIC SAMPLE

This consisted of 44 children in an orthopaedic ward whose
ages ranged from less than 1 year to eleven years old;
17 of the 44 were less than 5 years old.   Five of these
children were long-stay cases;   they all had severe

disabilities and the prognosis was poor. The remainder of the sample was admitted (generally to surgery), and discharged during the research project and varied considerably in the extent of impairment and previous hospital experience. The children came mainly from skilled working-class backgrounds and from households consisting of nuclear families.

The sample was categorised on the basis of health career (as defined earlier in this chapter) and the different patterns of hospitalisation the children had experienced (an aspect of treatment carrer). In Table 6.3 the categories are further sub-divided by age.

TABLE 6.3   The Orthopaedic Sample

Age (y)	A Long-term hospitalisation	B Admissions frequent throughout childhood	C Admissions for frequent plaster changes	D Limited previous experience	E No experience
0 to 2	2		5		2
3 to 4		2 severely impaired	1 moderately impaired 2 slightly impaired	3 slightly impaired	
5 to 10	3	3 seriously impaired 1 moderately impaired		3 moderately impaired 2 slightly impaired 5 unimpaired	7 unimpaired 3 slightly impaired
Total	5	6	8	13	12

(A) The long-stay children

All these children had been permanently in the hospital
since birth or early childhood and exemplify some of the
points made earlier in the discussion of the long-stay child.
One of the babies had been battered, the other belonged
to a gypsy family and had a condition leading to defective
muscle development. The mother had five other children
and they had moved on without any trace. Of the older
children one had been battered as a baby and the other two
were also severely impaired. One came from a single-parent
family where there were four other children, while in the
other case the mother kept up a very tenuous contact but
the father never came because 'he could not stand hospitals'.
    Because of their young age or the severity of their
impairment, four of the five children were unable to try
to control their interaction with nurses or to talk to the
others. The notable exception was the boy with no
communication difficulty. He had developed certain tactics
for dealing with the nurses, such as bargaining and invoking
Sister's authority, thus advancing a very limited measure
of self-determination. He also successfully interacted
with the other children passing through the ward by being
capable of sustaining a mutually rewarding relationship.
His comparative success in coping with the situation in
which he found himself may be attributed to the fact that
this was the setting in which all his previous formative
interaction had taken place. Unlike the other severely
handicapped children who were merely passing through, the
ward was his home. The friendliness and readiness to talk
which this boy exhibited would probably be interpreted by
those following the Bowlby approach as hiding an 'impaired'
capacity for warmth and constancy in relationships;
however, it is difficult to escape the conclusion that his
behaviour in the ward was socially acceptable to the staff
and, to that extent, he could be said to have adapted very
well to the situation in the ward as he found it.

(B) The severely impaired children with a history of frequent admissions

This consisted of the five most severely impaired children
in the sample and one classed as moderately impaired. All
had experienced a pattern of hospital admissions from early
childhood until the present in order to undergo corrective
surgery. On the whole these children had little or no
contact with peers outside school and when it came to
naughty behaviour and punishment, their parents tended to

adopt different standards for handling them compared with
their siblings. These variations were due to their
handicaps.

In the ward these children tended to have little contact
with other children and contact with the nurses only on
the nurses' terms. It is argued that this was because
they had few resources in the way of mobility and
communication skills to initiate and sustain interaction.
Despite their hospital experience there was little evidence
that they had learned appropriate techniques for obtaining
nursing attention or 'making out' in the ward. Lack of
control with other patients reflects their low hospital
interaction with peers and, in one case, inability to
sustain a friendly relationship with other children.

For example, one severely impaired boy used to attract
attention by pretending to fall out of bed or by balancing
dangerously on the locker or the traction apparatus and
shouting, 'Look at me!' The nurses' response was to
reprimand and scold and generally stigmatise him as a
troublemaker. He alienated the other children by hitting
them and taking their toys - tactics which broke the rules
of play and resulted in his exclusion from the main
groupings on the ward. Another moderately impaired boy
attempted to control the nurses by shouting abuse and
threats to them, unlike the other children who always made
legitimate requests, that is, legitimate in terms of the
ward culture. This had the predictable effect of making
the nurses less compliant and more punitive towards him.

After discharge these children showed less overall change
on the behavioural measures (8) than did children in the
other categories. This was partly because some of the
children were already so disturbed that little change was
noticed after this admission. Moreover, this admission
did not constitute the upheaval in the family life that it
undoubtedly did for some of the other children. The parents
had become accustomed to the child going to hospital and
to dealing with medical personnel. They appeared to have
come to terms with the problem of visiting and many of the
problems of handling severely impaired children at home.
They were the only category in which members had some
degree of outside help and support from social services
and voluntary organisations. The fathers' psychological and
practical support appeared to be of great value in helping
the mothers to cope. Naturally there were strains and
stresses and the parents were often worried about the
treatment and the pain and how the child would react.
But, on the whole, this was seen in a long-term perspective.
The parents were quite clear what they expected from the
child on discharge, and their real problems arose

not from this particular admission but from the long-term
prospect of dealing with a severely handicapped child. This
they had been doing since birth and in all cases appeared
to have developed some kind of philosophy and adjusted
their behaviour to cope with the situation.

(C) The very young children: recurrent admissions

These children had also been admitted from early childhood
but they are distinguished from the preceding category by
the fact that, after the first visit, the length of stay
is usually only for 48 hours to effect a plaster change.
These cases were generally congenital dislocation of the
hip and perthes disease, the prognosis was good and they
could expect to cease treatment with a cure completed.
The lives of these very young children had been dominated
by hospital. They had had little contact with other
children outside their own families and many were reported
as being shy of adult strangers.
   In the ward the youngest children in this category
had very little contact with other children. Their parents
were the main source of interaction, followed by the nurses.
This again was due to their limited communication skills,
lack of mobility and the fact that the children were
separated on an age basis. The older, more fluent,
members of the category were sometimes observed using
techniques to manipulate the nurses in a bid to get more
attention.
   After discharge, the children in this category were
much more likely to be reported by their mothers as
'clinging' and 'difficult to handle'. This was also
reflected in the large number showing increased
aggression after this admission. Separation anxiety was
by no means exclusive to this group since many older
children, particularly those who had not been in before,
also exhibited it. From the parents' point of view the
children's discharge did not result in a dramatic change
in the way they were handled since they had gone in with
plaster on and came out in the same state. The mothers
expected to do practically everything for these children.
   Problems arose when the other demands made by the family
also placed burdens on the mother, particularly if her
husband was not very sympathetic to her need for help.
Most received no help from outside the family although
there was evidence that one or two, at least, would have
welcomed some advice and help from a health visitor.
Running a home, dealing with other children and then having
to handle an immobile, clinging and aggressive child makes

considerable demands on a mother. The situation is not
helped if she cannot obtain the special equipment, such
as pushchairs, which enables the child to be taken out.
It is in these areas that the parents of such children are
most likely to face problems and need advice.

(D) and (E) Those who had some previous hospital experience
and those who had none

Category D consisted of all the other children in the
sample who had been in hospital before this particular
admission. This is rather a heterogeneous category,
containing children with differing health careers.
Category E was a residual one consisting of all those who
had no prior experience. All of them had regular contact
with their peers and the over-fives attended local primary
schools. There was some evidence that a couple of the
older children who were moderately impaired were becoming
aware of the stigma attached to physical imperfection.
However, this did not appear grossly to distort their
pattern of relations with other children. The parents
tended to treat all the children in both categories in
much the same way; the range of contacts, separation
experiences, expectations concerning help around the house
and handling of questions of discipline were virtually the
same.
     In the ward these children, the older ones anyway, had
the appropriate communication skills and ability to sustain
relations with peers, which enabled them to interact with
other patients. Some, at least, were likely to be mobile
at some point of their stay and this also gave them an
advantage when interacting. The presence or absence of
prior hospital experience appeared to make no difference
between the two categories with regard to the amount and
type of interaction they had with other children and the
nurses. The general pattern was high interaction with other
children and the utilisation of hospital equipment for
play purposes, combined with lower levels of interaction
with nurses. This was modified by the position of the
child in the ward and by the stage of treatment.
     Children from both categories were observed attempting
to gain nursing attention by various techniques. The most
sophisticated tactics for dealing with nurses were
observed among children whose health status would be
regarded as 'normal' (i.e. they had not suffered any
impairment until that time). This involved the establishment of identities as 'good patients' and attempts at
manipulation within the framework of ward rules. The ploy

of calling a nurse by her name was effective in getting
attention since it established a claim on her that was
difficult to ignore. Learning names and statuses is an
important part of beginning to structure the environment.
The shift system offered opportunities for exploring the
inconsistencies which could arise since one nurse did not
know what another had said or done. Summoning a nurse
using a perfectly legitimate reason as a pretext meant
that the child could maintain the identity of 'good patient'
while advancing her/his goal. This could most clearly be
seen in the matter of bedpans. Many of the children were
meant to be on their backs, thus very much restricting their
view of the ward. Use of a bedpan gave them a legitimate
reason for sitting up and taking stock of the situation.
Instances were observed in which children requested bedpans
very frequently and accosted each new nurse who appeared.

After discharge there was a difference between those
with prior hospital experience and those with none. The
under-fives who had not been in before were reported as
being more likely to exhibit general anxiety and repression
and greater apathy-withdrawal, whilst the over-fives were
more likely to show greater sleep disturbance. Those
who had been in hospital before showed more aggression,
and those whose previous admission had been reported by the
mother as resulting in disturbance were also more likely
to exhibit separation anxiety.

The loss of mobility entailed by discharge in plaster
was one of the major problems to which these children and
their families had to adjust. In the cases where this
occurred it represented a very big change and affected
relations within and outside the family. At one level the
child was less likely to have contact with peers and
became aware of her/his marginal status. At another level
the plaster meant that care had to be taken to avoid it
breaking down. This was difficult to avoid in travelling
to and from school. Pushchairs and wheelchairs were needed
for those who were not supposed to put any weight on their
feet and again there was some evidence of difficulties in
obtaining the right equipment. These parents face the
greatest disjunction between the child's state before and
after hospital. Although they may know that the child will
not be able to do much on discharge, the full implications
of the child's changed physical state and behaviour may
only become apparent in the weeks following the return home.
These parents again were given very little in the way of
advice or practical help to cope with the day-to-day
problems facing them.

CONCLUSION

This necessarily compressed account of the main findings
of our study serves to illustrate the potential of this
approach not only for research workers but, we would hope,
also for health administrators and professionals. Apart
from the actual findings, the categorisation in terms of
health-status and treatment-career variables highlights
a neglected group of child patients, namely the recurrent
admissions. The implicit dichotomy of the long-stay versus
the short-stay patient tends to obscure the fact that a
great many children have a history of admissions. The
implications of this have not in the past been fully
considered. Little is known about the long-term psychological effects of repeated admissions and there is no
evidence to suggest that this pattern is any less damaging
to a child's mental health than a stay involving months.
Parents are often not sure where to turn for advice
concerning management of the child and sometimes have
considerable difficulty in obtaining equipment. The
initiative is left entirely to them, and the hospital
appears to take little interest in the patient once
discharged, even though the child may be re-admitted in
the fairly near future. Within the broad category of
recurrent admissions further classification by health and
treatment variables helps us to understand why children
react to the ward in the way they do, and to make sense
of their parents' perceptions and reactions to them on
discharge.
     Finally it can be argued that the concept of health
status and the career perspective have much wider
implications. An attempt has been made to relate them
within the wider context of socialisation theory and to
indicate their potential with regard to other categories
involved with the child, particularly parents. These
concepts are not exclusively child focused, however, since
it seems possible to examine the interaction between
parents and doctors using their definitions of the child's
health status as an explanatory tool. It is suggested,
therefore, that health status might be given more attention
not only by medical sociologists but by sociologists
in general as an important variable in the study of
interaction.

CHAPTER SEVEN

On Calling for Order

Aspects of the organisation of patient care

David Hall

THE IMPORTANCE OF HOSPITAL ORGANISATION

In the series of research studies reported in this book an
underlying theme has been to uncover the reasons why
children appear to be vulnerable to a stay in hospital in
terms of behavioural disturbance, to construct a theoretical
explanation of such observations and to suggest ways of
overcoming such disturbance. Previous chapters have dealt
with children in hospital from a variety of perspectives
and have emphasised how consideration of children should
not be divorced from consideration of their family backgrounds or past experiences seen in terms of health and
treatment careers. But to deal with children in hospital
we shall have to adopt a further perspective and ask not
only how children respond to this environment but also how
the hospital works as a social organisation to treat sick
patients. To understand children's treatment we need to
understand the organisation of the hospital, for this will
affect children's activities in the wards. At the same
time we have to recognise that children are not just
passive respondents but will themselves cause changes in
the pattern of ward activities.

The early research at Swansea identified as important the
progression of a child from the home-centred system of
social relationships, to the hospital, characterised as a
qualitatively different system in that it is relatively
closed to outside influences and formally organised as a
place of work. The child then returned home, modified in
his behaviour by that hospital system (Stacey et al.,
1970, pp. 9-10). This model has guided further research
on the topic of children in hospital but, at the conclusion of the second phase of Swansea research, the
sociologists and psychologists who had worked from the
original model wished to refine the model on the basis of

their particular interests and research observations, in
order to bring out the parallels between their work (Hall,
Pill and Clough, 1976). What happened in the ward was
linked both to family interaction in the home and to the
attitudes and values of ward staff. It could now be
suggested that possibly too much emphasis had been placed
on the physical transference of children to the hospital
(and out again) in that this implied that family and
hospital were two separate and distinct social systems,
linked only by the admission and discharge of patients.
Although the authors of the earlier model would reject a
one-way view of socialisation, from teacher to the taught,
the impression given by the model was of children responding to environmental stimuli. The place of children
interpreting and giving meaning to the hospital situation
was not elaborated, nor were the actions of other
significant participants in the wards for the creation
and maintenance of ward environment.

PARTICIPANTS' PERCEPTIONS, DISCONTINUITY AND INTERACTION

In contrast an approach which is concerned with the subjective interpretation of perceptions, and its implications
for action, has been found to underlie much of what is
common in the theoretical aspects of the present research.
If we move the emphasis away from the physical aspects of
the hospital system and instead concentrate on the interpretation and understanding of such aspects by children, their
families and hospital staff, we shall be concerned with
the hospital/home dichotomy in so far as it is real for the
participants. For instance, the distinction may be emphasised by visiting regulations, or reduced by the introduction
of domestic play, and the social atmosphere of the ward
may more or less approximate to that of the home in
dimensions of warmth and proximity or of authoritarian or
democratic control.

By posing the relationship between home and hospital
in terms of a threatened continuity of experiences, we
would seek to posit a view of overlapping spheres of
influence, cross-cutting at the point of the child patient,
who in hospital may still retain strong social links with
his family but may find these becoming progressively
weaker as he becomes more accustomed and more skilled in
dealing with hospital-based relationships. The degree
to which various social systems converge on an individual
or, to put it the other way round, the degree to which an
individual orders his perceptions of the salience of
different relationships, will hold implications for his

actions. Loss of continuity, we argue, is stressful and
where such stress cannot be resolved, may give rise to
behavioural disturbance. This formulation, it can be
noted, is somewhat akin to that of multiple-role conflict,
which it has been proposed occurs when an individual is
called on to respond to contradictory expectations held
through possession of incompatible statuses. This has
been seen as a structural problem of social organisation,
which can be met by certain routinised and legitimated
avenues, such as the 'wearing of different hats' to avoid
conflicts of interests. But apart from the structural
features, role conflict too can be seen from an interactionist point of view in terms of the individual's
decisions about which roles to perform, and more
importantly, how to play those roles within the degree
of freedom allowed to, or claimed by, that person. In
reality, as Turner argues, simultaneous relationships with
others are not generally experienced as separate roles by
their enactors, so that 'what is inconsistent behaviour
viewed in relation to only a single type of relevant other
is perfectly coherent in relation to a system of others'
(1962, p. 30).

The whole context of interaction within hospital wards
is therefore relevant for an analysis of children's
behaviour. Essentially, the argument is for not merely
seeking how the child or individual responds to a situation,
but for exploring how he interprets, defines and acts on
his perceptions. I do not wish to abandon totally a
structural analysis; indeed, as I shall go on to show,
such an analysis of the hospital as an organisation can
add to our understanding of the problems of children in
hospital. Yet the link between social structure and
individual behaviour is problematic. What I wish to show
is a chain of causality and prediction between structure
and behaviour goes through individual perceptions, and that
we need to be able to understand how different people
interpret their situation. Applied to the hospital ward,
this means that on the one hand we recognise the spatial
barriers to communication with the outside world put up
by the four walls of the hospital, but that on the other
hand we allow for external influences to permeate those walls.

Even in Goffman's (1961) 'total institution', physical
separation is a necessary but not a sufficient condition
for behavioural modification, and it can be argued that
the type of control exerted is a more important factor in
changing attitudes and behaviour. Furthermore, it may
be argued that the type of control exerted within an
organisation is not independent of the norms of the wider
society in which that organisation is located, in that

from time to time it may be called upon to account for its exercise of power. This certainly is one conclusion that may be drawn from the series of hospital enquiries at Ely (DHSS, 1969) and afterwards: that although hospitals may in practice be for long periods unaccountable to the wider society and offer resistance to external investigation, they are ultimately responsible to public opinion for the exercise of their powers. There is an inherent tension between the self-closing aspects of the institution characterised as a private workplace, and the equitable treatment of patients as at the same time clients, consumers and work objects (Stacey, 1976).

HOSPITALS AS COMPLEX ORGANISATIONS

If we examine hospitals for the moment as complex organisations there is a number of points we can observe. We can identify sets of employees, typically organised in distinct hierarchies of rights and responsibilities; we may also identify sets of outcomes or goals to which the hospital, as any organisation, is working. Additionally we identify a set of clients, the patients, also participat- ing in the organisation. Their form of participation is, however, not as clear cut as it is for employees, for in terms of Parsons' pattern variables their involvement is usually the opposite of the affectively neutral, collectiv- ity oriented, universalistic, achievement-orientated and specific role prescribed for the doctor's relationship with patients (Parsons, 1951). Thus conflicts of interests can be predicted between staff dealing with patient X as a case of condition A, and patient X wanting consideration of himself as a unique individual. The response to this dilemma by some theorists has been to propose that doctors and nurses fulfil complementary roles in instrumental and expressive spheres respectively (Johnson and Martin, 1965), but the problem of the nature of their interaction with the patient is one faced by each occupation group in hospital.
The dissatisfaction of patients with the amount of information given to them by staff is well documented; it may be related not only to the structural imbalance between the involvement of staff and patients in the organisation, but may be an aspect of the control exerted by staff over patients (Waltzkin and Stoeckle, 1972). The practice of medicine is fraught with uncertainties, and in the course of their training doctors come to deal with this difficulty (Davis, 1960; Fox, 1975). Other studies in the communica- tion of diagnosis suggest that doctors tend to avoid premature disclosure by retaining to themselves the un- certainties of the situation, even beyond a point when

the element of doubt in their minds at least has been largely eliminated (Davis, 1963; West, 1977). This, it has been suggested, by Davis and Voysey (1975) is a way of dealing with a difficult situation when a diagnosis of a disability has to be communicated. Clough (1975) has also shown how knowledge of operations and their effects was carried by children in an orthopaedic ward, and that doctors considered the best way of imparting information was to allow children to find out the details from other children. Communication and control are important features of doctor-patient interaction, which may be linked with structural features of the hospital and consultation process whereby characteristics of interaction are influenced by the organisation of health care, and more particularly by the values which sustain the organisational arrangements.

With regard to the values that do operate, we find in hospitals - as in business organisations - a considerable difficulty in defining what actually are the values and goals towards which they work. What Is a Hospital For? is the title of an article by Sellors and Rains (1975), who plot the changing role of the hospital from sanctuary to workshop. An important element they note is the relationship between the hospital service and the community. In a cross-national survey, Glaser (1970) points to the relationship between societal values and the variations in the institutional form of hospitals, and suggests that non-technological variables derived from the external culture may create ambiguity and diversity in the goals and organisation of hospitals. The link between organisation and environment is familiar to those acquainted with such industrial studies as Burns and Stalker's 'Management of Innovation' (1961). The changing nature of the organisation is perhaps best illustrated by longitudinal historical studies, where developments are easier to isolate: Perrow (1963) provides an interesting example of the changing role of an American hospital based on changes in the environment and in the development of medical techniques, where changing relationships with the community were reflected in a different style of administration with greater control passing first to doctors and later to administrators.

The conclusion drawn from such studies is that organisations, or at least the members who constitute organisations, have numerous different goals which are pursued in various orders of priority. If we take, for example, as a single goal of a hospital, the healing of the sick, then it is a clear that such a goal cannot be attained in every instance. Studies of long-term or chronic wards (e.g. Coser, 1963) have pointed out how such a goal, if explicitly given as the purpose of nursing, may lead in Merton's (1957) terms to anomic responses of ritualistic or retreatist behaviour,

if the goal is incapable of fulfilment. Although with
children the likelihood of death in hospital is less, yet
the circumstance is then more difficult to accept, and we
found (Hall, 1977) that the aspect of children's suffering
and failure to recover was mentioned by many nurses as the
most difficult thing they had to deal with in hospitals.

AN INTERACTIVE APPROACH

While an analysis of the goals officially presented by
organisations may throw light on their ideologies and the
ways in which they seek public legitimation, as well as on
their pattern of internal structure, attention has tended
to be focused on how such goals facilitate co-operation
within organisations. The informal organisation of workers'
actions has often been considered to represent an alternative
form of co-ordination. It was then seen as a question for
research as to which form of organisation best achieved
the organisational goals and whether the method of goal
attainment had dysfunctional consequences. Such questions,
however, are invalidated if we accept the argument that the
formal inevitably exists with the informal, with both as
aspects of the relationship between individual and
organisation, between the search for predictability in
others and in the individual's capacity for improvisation
in role performance (see Goffman, 1971). This approach
follows Blumer's (1969) concern with symbolic interactionism, itself a development of Mead's formulations about the
'I' and the 'Me' (Strauss, 1956), or how an individual
experiences himself through the activities of others. This
perspective has been applied to hospitals, albeit mental
hospitals, by Goffman (1961) in his discussion of the moral
career of patients. He attempts to get at the meaning
assigned to their situation by patients, and their self-
evaluations, through the observed interactions of staff and
patients. Patient response, for Goffman, is something
created in the interplay between staff with their values
and objectives, and patients with theirs, where the outcome
may be either contributory or not contributory to the
organisation and its assumptions about patient behaviour
and identity. This interactive approach gives due weight
to staff as people who attempt either directly or indirectly
to fashion patient response, and it is to them that we
should now turn

RELATIONSHIPS AMONG STAFF

Some early research in mental hospitals (Stanton and
Schwartz, 1954; Caudill, 1958) had suggested that patient
disturbances could be provoked indirectly by conflict
among staff.   Coser (1976a) presents an extreme case
where suicides in a mental hospital are related to staff
morale.   However this might be, relationships among staff
are important for an understanding of ward activities in
all types of hospitals.   The hospital has attracted
attention from organisation theorists for its dual lines
of authority between medical and nursing staff, and the
tripartite system is completed by the administrative
section (Mauksch, 1973).   There are certain consequences
for the organisation of staff and for their attitudes to
work.   Nursing, for example, has been characterised in
terms of multiple subordination and blocked mobility,
raising the argument as to whether nursing can ever stand
as a profession equal to medicine or must be relegated
to a 'semi-profession' (Etzioni, 1969;   but see also Davies
and Francis, 1976).

The constitution and identity of professions has
attracted much sociological analysis, and medicine has been
seen as a particularly clear example of this form of work
organisation (Freidson, 1970).   The issue of professional
organisation affects not only the internal arrangements
of the medical profession but also its relationships with
other hospital staff, typically subordinate as paramedical
workers, and with patients.   The varying degrees of status
attached to different branches of medicine and their
pattern of segmentation have been discussed by Bucher and
Strauss (1960);   for the study of children in hospital,
this is of relevance to the standing of paediatrics in
comparison with other specialities.   An indirect measure
of the standing of paediatrics within medical specialities
in Britain is given by Stevens (1966) in her analysis of
consultants' merit awards.   Paediatrics comes towards the
middle of the ranking, neither highly over-represented
nor under-represented.   This may have some effect on the
overall distribution of resources within hospitals, and
indeed the moves to gather all children in hospital under
the care of paediatricians (Welsh Hospital Board, 1972)
has implications for the relative standing of different
branches of the medical profession as well as for the
levels of care given to patients.   The argument about the
emotional and behavioural disturbance of children in
hospital is a further reason for giving paediatricians
oversight of all children in hospital, on the grounds that
paediatricians are more likely to understand the problem
and take action to remedy it.

THE NURSES

It is with nurses, however, that the children are likely
to have greater direct contact, though this may only be
for a relatively small period of their time in hospital
(Hall and Cleary, 1974; Hawthorn, 1974). It is to nurses'
definitions of their work that we now turn. The arguments
about the status of nurses have been sketched above.
Much research has confined itself to the doctor-nurse-
patient triad, where the roles have been viewed as
complementary, but this simple analysis does not explain
the diversity and the pressures for change in the nurses'
role. On the one hand there is a move towards more
technical aspects of the work, shown in the USA by the
practice of the nurse-clinician, and in Britain towards
a managerial style of organisation following the Salmon
Report (Ministry of Health, 1966); on the other hand there
is a desire to return to basic skills at the bedside
defended in the Briggs Report (DHSS, 1972) and shown in
pressures for greater patient contact and disquiet about
the implications of the Salmon Report. Such problems in
the definition of the nurses' role, it can be argued, may
result in job dissatisfaction and have implications for
patient care.
    The problems of nurse-training have received much
attention, with concern being shown at the levels of
recruitment and wastage during and after training.
Research by Revans (1964) has shown correlations between
such organisational factors as staff turnover and
indicators of patient care such as length of stay. In
children's wards it is particularly relevant that three-
quarters of nurse-patient contact is made by nurses still
under training, who are in the wards as part of their
assignment and not by choice, and who may have no special
regard for children's problems, nor intend to pursue
children's nursing (Hall and Cleary, 1974; also Cleary,
chapter 5 above). Our study was designed to examine the
effects of introducing playleaders into children's wards,
and involved studies of children's activities before and
after playleaders started work. At the same time the
study provided an opportunity of investigating staff
attitudes to the playleader scheme and to their work in
general. This research has been presented in greater
detail elsewhere (Hall, 1977).

THE PARENTS

Although the doctor, nurse and patient are the main actors
in the interrelationships of the hospital process, with
children there are parents to consider as well. Pill
argues (chapter 6, above) that they constitute a most
important reference group in negotiating children's health
and treatment careers and in presenting the child to the
outside world. One interesting feature, therefore, to
arise out of the questionnaires administered to nurses by
both Fred Clough and myself was the strong negative view
of parents held by some nurses. When asked what the most
difficult thing about nursing children was, some nurses
replied bluntly: 'Parents', while other nurses consistently evaluated parents low on scales on instrumental
and expressive qualities. In part this may reflect the
difficulty of treating someone else's child with the parents
present, which seemed to cause the resistances to extending
parental visiting, which Pill (1967) noted and analysed
in terms of Goffman's (1971) distinction between 'back-
stage' and 'frontstage' in the presentation of self. The
reason why parents should be seen as hindrance rather than
the help which some of them were in serving meals and
attending to their children, is also related to the nurses'
own conceptions of their roles. Pill noted that nurses
were unwilling to let parents care for their children in
hospital, and Hawthorn (1974) found that ward sisters in
practice gave parents less responsibility than they said
they did. Some confirmatory evidence of the 'nuisance
value' of parents is given by Stimson (1976) from a
questionnaire survey of general practitioners, where
children accompanied by mothers were mentioned more
frequently as causing 'the most trouble' than children
by themselves.

OTHER STAFF

If parents constitute a particular problem for children's
wards, there are other participants in all wards who make
the doctor-nurse-patient triad untenable as a complete
model of the relationships existing on a ward. We have
also to consider those who go under the designation of
paramedical and ancillary staff. In the children's wards
we studied, our attention has been drawn to the activities
of the domestic staff and their relationships with the
other children, not only in directing children and maintaining order in the wards but also in restricting and
delimiting the scope of play activities. One should also

add physiotherapists, pathology technicians, ward
receptionists, and perhaps most interesting from an
organisation point of view, those professions external
to medicine but operating within the hospital: teaching
and social work. Play, too, is to some extent foreign to
the hospital, incorporating as it does both therapeutic
and educational goals. All of these illustrate relationships which are often forgotten when one concentrates on
the hospital purely as a curative institution, but all may
to different degrees affect a child's stay. Moreover, the
type of relationship between medical and nursing staff and
such other workers may be taken as evidence of the values
and attitudes held by doctors and nurses about the functions
and purposes of the hospital. As we have indicated above,
such notions may not be accepted equally by other
participants in the wards.

THE PATIENTS

Patients too must be considered as participants in the
wards. The Parsonian model of patient behaviour in the
sick role is typically submissive, with a common value
orientation between patient and doctor for working towards
the restoration of health. This model has been criticised
for failing to encompass the range of variety to be found
in the role and specifically by Bloor and Horobin (1975)
for relying on a medical orientation towards illness and
patient behaviour. Other specifications of patient roles
have suggested that a knowledge and power differential
operates between patient and doctor so that the role is
akin to that between child and parent, save that under
certain conditions the role may more closely approximate
to the relationship between adult and adult. One example
of the latter would be when the patient is suffering from
an incurable condition where the role of the doctor is
moderated from that of cure to one of support, and the
patient becomes an 'expert' in his condition. While such
an approach is useful in identifying different types of
patient role, it still maintains the assumption of control
over the situation being vested in the medical practitioner.
It could be suggested that there are times in the medical
encounter when the realities of control override the
assumptions, and patients are able to influence medical
decisions. Roth's (1963) observations of the structuring
of treatment decisions by patients, and Stimson and Webb's
(1975) analysis of the consultation in a doctor's surgery,
present a view of patients and doctors engaging in
tactical manoeuvres to put across their opinions. Thus

the direction of control cannot be assumed *a priori* for
any particular encounter, though the structural differential
between doctor and patient in terms of status and formal
position will enter into perceptions of the situation.
In the children's wards studied, instances were observed
when children, through familiarity with their own or their
neighbour's experience, possessed more knowledge about
technical aspects of their situation, such as the correct
way of using an inhaler for asthma, than some nurses
(often nurses in training and new to the wards). Clough
(1975) has noted how the 'old hands' among the children
carried a great amount of detail about treatment, which
on one occasion at least was passed on via a child who
had no personal experience of the treatment in question.
    Under examination the concept of the patient role breaks
down into a variety of different forms which express the
different sets of relationships encountered between staff
and patients. This, too, has consequences for a view of
the hospital as an instrument of socialisation and social
control. Taking the hospital as a form of 'people-
processing' organisation, patients can be seen in
organisational terms as a problematical input into the
system. They arrive as individuals but have to be treated
in standardised ways. The hospital seems to define what
behaviour is expected of patients and, characteristically,
according to Taylor (1970), seeks to impose more regulations
on patient behaviour than is absolutely necessary. The
corollary is that patients from time to time draw attention
to their view of the matter by sporadic refusals to conform.
It is not unreasonable to see hospitals as instruments of
socialisation, in that in treating patients they are also
engaged in creating an orderly environment. However, if
one concentrates on the organisational aspects of treatment
and the need for predictability in the system's input, one
is less likely to see non-conforming patient response as
rational action from the patients' perspective but more
inclined to dismiss it as irrational or positively wrong-
headed. A similar point about much of the literature on
the 'failure' of patients to follow prescribed medication
schedules has been made by Stimson and Webb (1975) in their
discussion of patients' interactions with doctors.
    The types of analysis which treat patients' communica-
tion or interaction as inadequate are suspect for the
reason that they adopt the standpoint of organisational
functionnaries without considering, for example, that such
organisations have no ultimate justifications other than
their clients, the patients. Yet in practice the
impression is sometimes given that patients tend to make
the wards 'untidy', and the tendency for nurses either to

appear busy or withdraw from the ward (Dodd, 1973) reflects
an ambivalence to including patients in the work of the
ward, which for children restricts the degree to which
nurses will play with them. The question of the relationship between type of patient and form of hospital
organisation is an interesting one that has been considered
by Rosengren and Lefton (1969). They argue that the type
of patient treated has many implications for the organisation of the institution, and not just for the type of
socialisation procedures employed but also for the values
and attitudes of staff, as shown in such items as readiness to innovate. They argue that hospitals may be
classified according to the extent and degree of involvement they have with the patient, thus distinguishing
short- from long-stay hospitals, and distinguishing those
which care for all aspects of a patient's welfare from
those concerned with a specific part or condition only.
They postulate that the quick-repair, quick-return hospital
is only minimally susceptible to ideological as opposed
to technical innovation.

While this approach is useful in distinguishing types
of hospitals by integrating consideration of the patient
with specification of organisational forms and processes,
it still fails to explain the sources of variation within
hospitals of similar types. In placing the main determinants of organisational character with the patient intake,
it provides only a monocausal explanation for what is a
complex problem. Pill has shown (in chapter 6) how the
distinction between short- and long-stay hospitals is
primarily a matter of administrative decision, and the
increasing trend towards more frequent and shorter stays
for long-term conditions is obfuscating this distinction.
Moreover, our joint experiences in short- and long-stay
wards suggested that the immediate problems for children
were much the same, though the long-term effects may vary.
Although we were unable to test the hypothesis about
differential sorts of innovation, it would appear that
change in either environment would not be easy.

SOCIAL CONTROL

One theme which runs through the analysis offered so far,
whether we view it from a concern with socialisation or
from a concern with patterns of interaction, is that of
control. Organisations, as forms of co-ordination,
necessarily revolve around issues of control, whether for
the setting and achievement of internal arrangements or
external goals. In organisations certain forms of control

are commonly legitimated by participants and accepted as a
means of carrying out the business of the organisation;
but a concern with interaction in organisations shows that
such legitimacy is not unproblematical and that in practice
the issue of control is potentially always under debate
in one aspect or another. It is this divergence between
formal analysis and the results of observations at various
points within organisations that illustrates the
deficiencies of assuming power to be constant. Etzioni's
(1961) classification of types of control and of participants' commitment to the organisation is well known, and
his analysis of the general hospital as a normative
organisation is helpful in showing what kinds of orientation one might predominantly expect within hospitals. But
this overall classification must necessarily obscure the
many other kinds of power relationships existing at ward
level. For example, although it could be argued that
normative involvement of staff has been used to depress
wages and salaries, it is clear that the economic arguments
and utilitarian involvements are now coming to the fore.
At ward level, in the relationships between nurses and
patients we found that direct methods of control, of a
rather coercive nature, were fairly high on the power
options chosen by staff when dealing with child patients,
where their physically small size and weight were not
unimportant aspects of how they were perceived by nurses.
     If the hospital is not completely a normatively run
organisation, nevertheless there are aspects when hospital
staff may act to impose their values on the situation as
'moral entrepreneurs'. In their emphasis upon children's
obedience in the wards, nurses were inclined to attribute
naughtiness to the child who had been 'spoilt' by his
parents. On a wider level Voysey (1975) argues for the
medical explanation of disability as forming a modern
legitimation for such conditions in the wake of the decline
of the acceptability of religious legitimations, and
analyses medical practice in this instance as fashioning
and to some extent imposing definitions of normality. In
doing so, she argues, medical legitimations compel parents
to present an outward appearance of normality, of coping
as well as can be expected. The argument has been stated
in its broadest form by Illich (1975), and by Zola (1975b)
under the heading of the medicalisation of everyday life,
drawing attention to 'the expansion of those areas of
life deemed relevant to the good practice of medicine'.

WHERE POWER LIES

Besides the more general aspects of the dominance of
medical legitimations in everyday life, we may also focus
on the distribution and management of power within hospitals.
In doing this we find a pattern not as clear cut as that
seen from above, where doctors and in particular consultants hold the greater power. The power of the consultant
has been analysed by Davies (1972), and while we must agree
that the consultant is able to initiate new programmes of
medical and social care in the wards it is also evident
from many hospital studies from Belknap onwards (see
Perrow, 1965) that the formal authority of the consultant
does not necessarily extend all the way down to the ward
floor.
      One of the reasons for this lies in the previously
noted separation of powers between medical, nursing and
administrative staffs; but also important is the place
that ward activities take in the consultant's scale of
priorities. Typically, the consultant spends a limited
amount of time in the ward at ward rounds, which have a
formal, even ritualistic, tradition attached to them. For
one consultant, all parents in a children's ward were
asked to leave the ward during his rounds. Consultants
see the publicly presented face of the ward, and tend not
to see the interactions among other staff in the ward.
Even if they do, they are likely to consider it as the
ward sister's responsibility, not their own, which is
restricted to supporting her authority. In a study of
perceptions of an actual and an ideal ward, Clough found
that of hospital staff it was the consultant who thought there
was the greatest similarity between the ward as it actually
existed and the ward as it ideally should be.
      Perceptions of the ward, then, vary at different levels
in the hierarchy; and so, too, does the exercise of power
in maintaining order. Using a replication in the children's
wards of a technique for measuring nurses' power orientations, an interesting range of opinions was found. While
the predominantly preferred response was one of 'benevolent
manipulation', that is, getting children to act through
indirect pressure, thus confirming the earlier findings
(Rosenberg and Pearlin, 1962), it was noticeable that
nurses did differ in their ranking of power options, such
that some placed higher priority on direct methods of
command or coercion, while some stated they would opt for
a laissez-faire choice, that is, to do nothing and let
children get away with bad behaviour. The result of this
enquiry was to show that the predominant mode of response
was not universal but had wide variations, with the

implication that there was no clear policy on dealing with
disruptive children but that each nurse followed her own
inclination. The result was likely to be an inconsistent
pattern of control, bearing in mind the number of different
nurses that dealt with a child each day. An inconsistent
pattern of control, it may be hypothesised, will be much
more difficult for a child to come to terms with, and
cause more anxiety and disturbance, than a settled and
predictable order, whether democratic or authoritarian in
essence.

Inconsistencies in control are also shown in the tension
between the legitimate use of authority in furthering
co-ordination among participants towards the achievement
of common goals, and the use of power by groups or
individuals to achieve limited personal ends, including the
performance of their work without interference from others.
It is a matter for debate how far all control other than
coercion rests in the willingness of those subject to it
to conform (see Blau, 1964); authority and power in the
sense used above are engaged in a continuous dialectic
when we come to examine working relationships at ward level.
The instance of the cleaners in a children's ward is a
particularly vivid example, where power resided in people
who in formal terms had little authority but who were able
to use their position to mobilise traditional values of
cleanliness and order to their advantage, and to determine
how others should fit in with them. The power of lower
participants has been analysed by Mechanic (1968), and
the relationship between domestic and play staff has been
discussed in detail elsewhere (Hall, 1977).

The conclusion of this short discussion about power
and control is to say that the topic is one of great
relevance both to the constitution of organisations such
as the hospital and to the interactions of participants,
such as staff and patients. We have found the need to
distinguish between the power of individuals to operate
at different levels with the organisation - for example,
with consultants at hospital policy level and on the ward
floor - and also to distinguish among similar participants
at the same level, as in the inconsistency of nurses'
power orientations. Power can be seen not so much as an
independent variable given by position in the organisation
(though formal rights and responsibilities do provide a
framework for action) but rather as a potentiallity for
control exerted through interaction at all levels, and
changeable with shifting balances and alliances.

NEGOTIATED WARD ORDER

To return to the ward, we see it not so much as a social
structure constituted according to a prescribed pattern,
though obviously this is one element in the situation,
but as a field or arena for interaction among staff and
patients. It is the interaction which serves to set
limits to, and define, what the ward is, how it is perceived by each of the participants. This approach owes
much to Strauss et al. (1963), who put forward the concept
of 'negotiated order' to explain their observations in
wards of a psychiatric hospital. They started from a
point of seeing the rules and regulations of the hospital
were not immutable, and that the hospital, although having
the appearance of a rule-bound institution, was in reality
much more flexible. This occurred because the rules were
selectively applied, being enforced for particular
instances at particular times to meet current problems,
and then lapsing into disuse as the immediate problems
changed. Our own observations have shown the uncertainty
and ambiguity arising among staff in their dealings with
children, and have raised the maintenance of order,
predictability and control as key issues.

Attention, therefore, was turned to the processes
whereby agreements or priorities came into being through
the interaction of those in the wards. To Strauss and
his associates the hospital was not the formal institution
but the sum of regulations, agreements and understandings
operating at any time. Such a view, however, has to be
integrated into a perception of the hospital containing
certain less easily changeable elements, which the notion
of formal organisation was intended to capture. While
it may be true that in the long term, all rules are
negotiable, any practical study is faced with discovering
that certain rules are less changeable than others, and
it is these that can be seen as lending a framework, albeit
a moving one, to everyday interaction. Silverman (1970)
comments on the relationship between an observer's
research perspective and his view of organisation by noting
that: 'to ask what is the role-system of an organisation
is to freeze ongoing interaction at one single moment in
time'.

However, the concept of negotiated order does direct
our attention to the processes observable in the ward, and
provides a way of linking individual activity with the
sharing or imposing of common perspectives on values. To
what extent can there be a common perspective between staff
and patients? Theoretical formulations of patient and
staff roles would posit that there is a common perspective

oriented around a common goal of cure, while empirical
observations suggest that the commonness of that perspective is often illusory, and that individuals hold complex
and sometimes mutually conflicting views of their situation
in terms of multiple rather than single rationality.
Clough's analysis (chapter 3, above) of the meaning of
hospital, illness and treatment is one example.

MEMBERS AND OUTSIDERS

The sociological observer, it should not be forgotten,
faces similar problems of creating order out of his perceptions and experiences. Particularly if the observer
has no medical qualifications, he may find on entering
a ward that his own perceptions are closest to those of
the patient, in seeing things with fresh eyes. It could
be argued that lack of medical qualification may result
in a tendency to ignore illness and concentrate too much
on social relations; but in contrast it should be noted
that medical and nursing staffs themselves have only a
partial view of what goes on in the ward as a consequence
of their work, as Hawthorn (1974) found when she required
nurse tutors to act as sociological observers in children's
wards, and they then saw things they had not seen as nurses.
Such experiences lend greater weight to the arguments in
favour of playleaders in children's wards, as people who
are not tied to nursing duties but have the time and
opportunity through extended contact with children to
represent their interests and alleviate their anxieties.
In so far as the hospital does constitute a system with
its own medical meanings, patients form a class of
'outsiders', to which the observer will probably belong
until he stays long enough to begin to acquire knowledge
of these other meanings.
    The distinction between the 'closed' organisation of
the hospital and the 'outside' orientation of patients
gives some validity to the view of patients and hospital
staff constituting separate and enclosed worlds. Such a
distinction is relative, however, given the degree of
patients' and staff's experience and involvement through
health and illness careers. As we have seen, some patients
may become more 'at home' in the wards than some staff.
A major problem for new patients, however, will be with
the strangeness of the ward, and a predominant feature of
that strangeness will be uncertainty about what is
happening or is about to happen, and when they will be
able to go home. The importance we found attached by
children to their beds as a thing 'most liked' about

hospital can perhaps be attributed to its place as the
child's base in the ward.   It was noticeable that at
visiting times in the children's wards parents used to
take their children from where they happened to be in the
wards and return to the child's bedside to conduct their
visiting there.   After the opening of the playroom this,
too, was used for visiting.   Brown's finding of a correlation between parental visiting and increased immobility
of the child (chapter 2) may then be an outcome of spatial
allocation to parents in the wards.   In part, parents could
be seen to be deferring to staff's expectations of a tidy
presentation of the ward for inspection by visitors;   but
also, the observations showed how parents were looking for
a place to which they could be certain of having a legitimate claim and that was the bedside and later the
playroom.   People attempted to structure the uncertainty
by applying or constructing rules for procedure on the
basis of what they knew about hospital procedure or thought
would be acceptable to the hospital staff.

PROBLEM-SOLVING

In general, the activities of participants in the wards
could be seen as forms of problem-solving, where they
attempted to develop an agreed basis for interaction on
the grounds of their own experience and expectations of
others' activities.   While the problem-solving perspective
is most readily applicable to the activities of patients
and their parents, it can equally be argued that patients
represent a problematic and varying input into the hospital,
so that staff have to engage in problem-solving behaviour.
Furthermore, when changes are introduced into wards, as
with the experimental introduction of playleaders, the
activities of all participants involve problem-solving.
Indeed the nature of the problem is also an aspect which
is worked out through interaction between the different
participants, in that with playleaders, for example, what
their work consisted of was to a large measure constrained
by what they were allowed by others to do.
     This perspective of problem-solving involves the
perception of a given situation in the light of relevant
past experiences or values orienting towards future action,
and worked out through interaction and the response or
anticipated response of others.   It is a perspective drawn
from symbolic interactionism, which nevertheless has
parallels with the models developed above about balance
theory, discontinuity and persistence, and the subjective
interpretation of career.   It is on the basis of these

parallels that we argue for the closer integration of different research perspectives in examining observed behaviour in the hospital and the home, and in throwing light upon the complexities of the observed situations, and their meanings for those involved.

CHILDREN'S DISTRESS IN HOSPITAL AND AFTER

So far, we have concentrated on showing how an analysis of the hospital as a complex organisation is relevant to any discussion of patient behaviour, and how staff and patient interactions are important determinants of what the hospital actually is. It is time now to bring the discussion back to the problems of children in hospital, with which the whole programme of research originated. The question of children's vulnerability to a stay in hospital still remains, though now we have indicated how maternal deprivation and the effects of illness are qualified by the strangeness of the situation and the degree to which children (and others) are able to perceive and understand events around them. A part of that strangeness is contributed by the uncertainty children feel about what is going on, and what they should do. The frequently noted succession of caretakers in hospitals, which has previously been linked to factors of maternal deprivation and multiple mothering, may equally be seen as increasing confusion and uncertainty. It results in a situation where different nurses have been observed to issue conflicting instructions to children, and where children who are not readily articulate find it difficult to communicate their needs to each member of staff who takes care of them.

Clarke and Clarke (1976) have cast doubt upon the relationship found between early hospital stay and later behavioural disturbance, suggesting that both hospital admission and disturbance are symptoms of pre-existing family and environmental disadvantage. Nevertheless, the short-term distress and disturbance caused by hospital treatment is supported by research findings; and it remains to be seen whether improvements to the hospital as an institution can eliminate disturbance within hospitals, though the results of employing playleaders provide limited grounds for optimism. It would be unfortunate if debate about the aetiology of long-term disturbance were to direct attention away from those features of hospital treatment which produce immediate distress and are amenable to analysis and to remedial action.

CHILDREN'S RESPONSES TO UNCERTAINTY

A basic concern in this chapter has been to suggest how
an understanding of the organisation of the hospital and
the values and attitudes of those involved may prove to
be an alternative way of analysing the interaction of
children in hospital, in distinction from theories of
maternal or environment deprivation. By focusing on the
meaning that actors ascribe to the situation, we set the
ground for examining the activities of doctors, nurses,
paramedical staff, auxillary staff and parents as equally
problematical as those of children.

Applied to the child patient, the model of children
making sense of uncertainty offers a rather different
interpretation of the so-called 'settled' behaviour of
children in hospital which Robertson (1970) has noted
as a disturbed state. The notion here would be that
withdrawal is a rational and congruent response to a
system of care which puts an emphasis on obedience, on
lack of noise, and in which the child who gets the most
attention is the one who creates the most disturbance, while
the quiet child tends to be ignored (see Pill, in Stacey
et al., 1970, p. 109). Disturbance then lies in the
difficulties of re-adaptation to a different environment
outside the hospital after reaching an accommodation to
the situation within. Thus the emphasis is placed not
merely on the different situations applying in the home
and the hospital but on the abilities of individuals to
adapt their perspectives to change.

ATTEMPTS AT AMELIORATION: PLAYLEADERS

The basis for attempts to ameliorate the position of
children in hospital has been that of altering the hospital
environment to be more near to that of the home. Thus
maternal deprivation has been countered by pressure for
increased parental visiting and, for young children at
least, mother-and-baby units. These changes have been
accepted slowly in many hospitals, and in one of those
studied at least the mother-and-baby unit was almost
continuously occupied by children only. Following from
the difficulties of mothers unable or unwilling to stay
in hospital with their children, playleaders have been
suggested for children's wards. While the idea may have
originally been of a mother-substitute (and the ward-
granny scheme (Jolly, 1975) now develops this idea), the
direction of play leadership has turned much more towards
education and therapy but still with the aim of replicating

a normal nursery/home environment within the hospital. My own research has looked at play in hospital with an educational component and has found that it counteracts the tendency of children to stay immobile and inactive in bed by increasing their opportunities for activity and interaction. Playleaders are greatly liked by children, and they are able to work at a continuous personal level with children, whether it be to comfort children and assist nurses during treatment, or simply to explain what is going on to children and interpret their wishes to staff. I see the role of playleader not so much as mother-substitute but rather as the child's representative.

It remains to be seen whether different styles of play leadership would have different effects on children, and in particular how successfully they would be able to prepare children to cope with the discontinuity between home and hospital.

This approach suggests a more flexible method of operation than fitting the hospital to suit the home, if only for the simple fact that home environments vary greatly. Our study indicated that children from an authoritarian family background were rated by their mothers as worse rather than better after hospital. This may have been due to their background unfitting them for dealing with the laissez-faire ambiguities of the ward. However, the earlier data of Dearden (in Stacey et al., 1970, p. 83) give no support to this particular finding, so the corre-spondence between home and hospital environment, and its effects on children's behaviour, must as yet remain undetermined. The authority structure of the wards involved may be an important variable.

Whether or not adaptability to change is relevant to children's disturbance, it is certainly relevant to a study of staff's response to innovation, and in particular to the introduction of playleaders. I have argued that what the playleader was able to do, in effect the deter-mination of her role, was strongly influenced by the con-tinuing sequence of her interactions with other participants in the ward. Among these were some who were resistant to change for a variety of reasons, and who were able to manipulate the shared values of other staff, for instance, towards order and tidiness as essential elements in hospital administration and the healing process, to impose limits on what the playleader might do. I have analysed the predominant reaction of staff to this innovation as one of detachment and isolation, whereby each continued working as before with minimal concessions made to the new member of the ward staff, implying an unwillingness to adapt existing views

of what her work should be. The result was a certain
amount of role conflict for playleaders and other staff,
and ultimately some degree of failure to achieve the
benefits which might be expected from play in hospital.

HOME OR HOSPITAL TREATMENT?

Given the magnitude and complexity of the problem of
children's disturbance both during and after a spell in
hospital, which has been shown in numerous studies in
addition to the Swansea programme of research, and also
given the limited success of schemes such as parental
accompaniment or playleaders in combating such disturbance,
we must question whether in fact the hospital is the best
place for treating sick children. Although this question
might appear to be a radical and perhaps idealistic
contribution to the debate about the welfare of children
in hospital, it is worth noting that it has been put before -
and by the Platt Committee Report of 1959 (Ministry of
Health, 1959). There it was argued that in view of the
evidence that had accumulated on children's disturbance,
admissions should be avoided if at all possible. While the
committee saw this recommendation as a means of drawing
off those children most likely to succumb to a hospital
experience, the broader question inevitably follows of
whether hospitals *per se* are suitable for the treatment
of patients (and not just younger children). If not, why
not? The answer to this second question,I have suggested,
lies in a consideration of the processes operating within
a hospital as a consequence of it being a complex organisation with many groups of participants, each to some extent
with conflicting interests. Duff and Hollingshead, on
the basis of their study in an American hospital, also
point to the lack of direct and effective control over
the care of patients, and particularly the personal aspects
of that care. They pose the question: 'Can physicians
treat disease in the perspective of patient and family
realities, or are they capable of treating disease only
in a more abstract sense?' (Duff and Hollingshead, 1968,
p. 379).
     With respect to young children, I have argued that
playleaders are an important element in helping 'to
interpret the hospital to the child and the child to the
hospital' (quoted in Hall and Cleary, 1974), and so
furthering a mutual understanding of others' problems.
By insisting on care for all aspects of a child, and in
particular the child's emotional and cognitive development,
playleaders also constitute to some degree a different

model for treating patients in hospital from the purely
medical model of treating diseases. The opposition between
medical treatment of disease and concern for the patient's
perspective is illustrated by Glaser's (1970) international
survey, and summed up in his proposition that the more
widespread family care of sick members in hospital is,
then the weaker are the hospital's controls over patients
and the greater is its responsiveness to the patient's
conception of treatment.

If we take seriously the difficulties of providing such
treatment within the orthodox ward environment, it is
instructive to see how these might be lessened - for example,
by paediatric home nursing. This has been applied in
several areas in Great Britain, with results that appear
encouraging (Oppé, 1971). However, their wider application
rests on local conditions, and the success of such schemes
will depend, as does that of playleaders, on the extent
to which such alternative procedures are accepted into
the full range of medical services. Certain demographic
changes, such as the increasing prevalence of married
women working and of single-parent families, will limit
the extent to which home-based treatment can be substituted
for hospital care. Even should such substitution be
possible, we must still ask whether the family itself is
indeed always the most suitable environment for treating
the sick child. The substance of recent criticisms of
the maternal-deprivation model (e.g. Clarke and Clarke,
1976) has been to re-examine the family as being necessarily
the best environment for young children, by challenging
the dictum that has arisen of 'Any home better than no
home', and to question whether the family is not rather
a repressive set of relationships (Coser, 1976b).

This is not the place to develop the argument any
further, except to express the hope that future consideration of children's response to hospital will explore in
greater detail the overlapping of the social systems
of hospital and family. In the last resort, questions
about the best environment for children, for hospital
patients and for hospital staff, rest on value judgments
where agreement will perhaps always be less than perfect.
Nevertheless, just as King, Raynes and Tizard (1971)
declared their belief that child-orientated management
practices are 'better' for children than institutionally
oriented practices, so I would wish to echo their statement as to the qualities I think should be preferred
in the care and treatment of children in hospital.

CONCLUSION

The purpose of this chapter has been to explore the world
of the hospital and to suggest that it has not been paid
sufficient attention as a special case of social relationships which involve and affect children's activities. We
would argue that consideration of children's response to
hospital cannot be divorced from consideration of that
environment as a social system, constituted and reconsti-
tuted by the pattern of encounters among participants.
The problem of children in hospital is a complex one which
admits of no simple solution but where a number of
different perspectives can contribute their own special
understanding of aspects of the problem, resulting both
in additions to a theoretical model and in practical
recommendations for action.

In terms of changes to hospital procedures,
recommendations for the increased use of playleaders are
likely to be turned down at times of financial stringency
(DHSS, 1976), but the experience of using playleaders
shows that one basic problem is the disparity of values
between playleaders and other hospital staff which can
limit the playleaders' role. It is arguable that as long
as such a disparity exists, the mere fact of the employment
of playleaders will not change staff's attitudes to the
treatment of sick children. Given the comparatively short
experimental period of our study - six months - we are
unable to say whether a change of attitudes might occur
over a longer period, though there are indications in the
subsequent response to the research report by staff in the
hospitals that this may be so.

One practical conclusion from this study is that non-
costly measures should, and must, also be used if the
treatment of children in hospital is to change. In our
report to the Department of Health we recommended that
much more attention should be paid to the reduction of
uncertainty and ambiguity for children on the ward and to
maintaining continuity of care; also that parents should
be given greater information about hospital procedures
and actively involved in the care of their children in
hospital; that all grades of staff should be chosen with
due regard for their understanding and sympathy for
children; and that greater training should be given to
nurses and other staff in the emotional and educational
needs of children. If these things were to be done we
would have greater confidence in the ability of all staff
to understand the problems of children in hospital, and of
the possibility of attacking the original problem of the
welfare of children in hospital.

CHAPTER EIGHT

The Practical Implications of our Conclusions

Margaret Stacey

INTRODUCTION AND OVERVIEW

Our concern in this volume has been with child patients, not simply with paediatric patients, for our concern is with children rather than with paediatrics as a speciality. Child patients are to be found in many parts of the hospital and not always in situations where the paediatrician has oversight. Increasingly since the Platt Report (Ministry of Health, 1959) children have been gathered together in children's wards under paediatricians but many are still to be found elsewhere: in ENT wards, in eye wards, in general surgery.

There is also the question of the age range. In some children's wards patients are deemed too old for the ward at 8, though most frequently children from about 12 years onwards are admitted to adult wards. The Welsh Hospital Board Working Party (1972), taking all ages under compulsory school leaving age as a rule-of-thumb definition of 'child', found that from two-thirds to four-fifths of children in hospital were under the care of specialists other than paediatricians. The Court Report does not include a table showing to which wards or under which specialists children are admitted but it does suggest that half the children admitted to hospital are admitted for surgery ' and the major part of this is done by general or specialist surgeons whose main work is with adults' (para. 18.26); that almost as many children of school age are admitted to orthopaedic as to paediatric beds (para. 18.35); that the same is true for otolaryngology and audiology (para. 18.36); and 1 patient in 5 in departments of ophthalmology is a child (para. 18.37). Experience in the Welsh Hospital Board area suggested that greater concern was expressed for the all-round needs of children in paediatric wards rather than in other wards. The large number treated elsewhere is therefore of particular note.

Taking children as a whole, the large proportion experiencing hospital nowadays has also to be borne in mind.   By the age of 7 some 45 per cent of children may have been admitted to hospital (R. Davie et al., 1972), and each year about 6 per cent of children are admitted to hospital (DHSS, 1976b, para. 12.37).

While in our first round of studies we looked specifically at pre-school children, in this round we have spanned infancy to adolescence, for it follows from our approach that we do not believe that psycho-social understanding of the child patient should be limited to the pre-school years.   In view of the large numbers of children outside paediatric departments it is appropriate that our studies should have covered children in paediatric, ENT and orthopaedic wards, for these wards represent something of the range experienced by children in hospital.   We have no examples of eye wards, nor have we looked at the situation for children in adult wards, but we have had available to us the results of a survey of children in hospital in all situations undertaken for the Welsh Hospital Board (Stacey and Earthrowl, 1973).

We do not claim that our wards are in any statistical sense representative of all wards.   We do believe that the kinds of social relations we have looked at are typical of the ward experiences of staff and child patients.   Indeed, as Hall has pointed out in the introduction to this volume, we believe that many of our findings are relevant to other categories of patient also.   We claim that our findings are typical of the ward experience of staff and child patients because many of the features that we believe dominate the relationships we have observed are inherent in the typical organisation of medicine and of hospitals as such.   We are further encouraged in this view by the consonance between our findings and those of others working in quite different situations (Hawthorn, 1974;   Harrisson, 1974).   There are a few hospitals where deliberate and major attempts have been made to modify the character of a ward and where our findings might not, therefore, apply in a general sense, but these wards are not typical.   In so far as these wards are often cited as examples of best practice it may not be easy for leaders of medical opinion and administration to remember the average practice of the average or below average NHS hospital, especially those in the less advantaged parts of large cities or in the less advantaged regions.   Despite attempts to encourage uniformity the range of performance of NHS hospitals is wide (Stewart and Sleeman, 1967).

If health-care professionals have not found our accounts

emotional and cognitive aspects of their patients than are
some other specialists. In *Paediatrics in the Seventies*
there are few references to the specific hazards of
separation for the young, or of the strange situation of
the hospital, or of the trauma of illness or treatment.
The matter is raised in the introduction of that book,
where it is advised that mothers should come into hospital
with pre-school children on the grounds, among others, that
'even if the long-term effects of separation are less
severe than was at first suggested, joint admission is
biologically natural (sic)'. Where mothers cannot come
in with their children 'free visiting is a second best,
and this should be normal practice with older children'
(p. 9). The matter is not referred to again except to
support the arguments for day care (p. 31), and with
regard to children with malignant diseases in regional
centres (p. 56).

The Court Committee showed a lively awareness of social
epidemiology, of social factors in the causation of
illness, but showed little appreciation of the importance
of the social organisation of health care, the social
relations among professionals and between professionals
and patients. The relevance of administrative organisation is appreciated as are the more technical aspects of
the division of labour, but the sociological aspects are
imperfectly recognised. Where recognition is given to
these factors they are not systematically conceived
(DHSS, 1976b).

Common sense and social science

Most of the social arrangements found in hospitals, where
they do not derive directly from hospital practice or
procedure, have their roots in common sense or common
culture. Access to seriously ill or dying children has
long been accorded. This derives from cultural expectations about behaviour towards the dying and not specifically
from social science. Another procedure which seems to
derive entirely from folk culture and not from research
findings is the segregation of children from adults.
Where all children cannot, for whatever reason, be nursed
in a children's ward with children's facilities it is
deemed more appropriate to nurse them in a cubicle on
their own than among adults. The Platt Committee
(Ministry of Health, 1959) thought that the sights and
sounds in an adult ward were inappropriate for children.
Because of that committee's stress on the mother-child
unit, little thought was given to separation and

strangeness as such. Yet it is arguable that a child
would find it more traumatic being alone in a single
cubicle than he/she would in an open ward with adults,
some of whom might choose to play a surrogate-kin role.
The policy which encourages the withdrawal of children to
single-bed cubicles has nothing to do with research
findings about separation, strangeness or adult company,
but reflects the feelings of adults about what idealised
children ought to feel when faced with adult illness and
suffering. The policy also reflects notions of segregation
based on age-grading, common in our society, especially
in middle- and upper-class homes (Newson and Newson, 1965;
Bronfenbrenner, 1970).

It is interesting that alone among scientific social-
science research findings the Bowlby hypothesis has
received wide acceptance. The notion that separation in
hospital may be harmful to young children is now
generally accepted by paediatricians and some other
consultants and by increasing numbers of nursing and other
caring staff. James Robertson and John Bowlby must take
a good deal of the credit for the change in professional
and public attitudes to the treatment of children in
hospital. Robertson's evidence presented to the Platt
Committee was widely disseminated and read thereafter.
The Bowlby-Robertson hypothesis, like the more recent
expositions of Bianca Gordon (Gordon, 1973, 1974) is based
initially on the notion of the mother and child as a
biological unit: initially, at least, separation does
physical violence because it does biological violence.
The biological base partly explains why psychoanalytic
theory which stresses the dangers of separation of mother
and child appeals to some doctors. One of the most
important scientific bases of medical training is the
biological and it is understandable that explanations
which relate to biological should have a salience and
therefore a credibility for doctors. Indeed in *Paediatrics
in the Seventies,* as indicated above, the biological model
tends to be used for all social explanations. Similar
explanations underlie the social epidemiology of the
Court Committee (DHSS,1976b).

It is not surprising that this should be so. Medical
practitioners are trained to look at people predominantly
in terms of a biochemical model. The concepts of psychology go beyond the biochemical model but are based on it.
Psychology, generally speaking, relates to the individual
organism. This is an approach which makes reasonable sense
to clinicians because their concern is to treat individual
organisms. The sociologist looks at people, of course,
but the units with which the sociologist deals are more

than this. The sociologist is concerned with groups, with
people in interaction, with shared beliefs and feelings.
The mother-child relationship, with its biological base,
is easy to grasp, so is the family. The great majority
of sociological entities, however, have no biological base
in that sense - for example, a hospital, a ward, a friendship, a social institution. Our case is that the social
experiences of the child as well as her/his psychological
experiences are central to successful therapy, and that
therapy itself is a social action, and therefore that all
those concerned with health care must come to terms with
and assimilate a sociological approach.

Illness, treatment and suffering

Those who have read the chapters by Brown and Clough will
have become aware that the psychological cannot be understood without reference to the sociological. In Brown's
work the social arrangements which had been experienced
in the family, and the child's behaviour in that context,
were directly relevant to the way in which the child
experienced hospital and her/his reactions to it. In
Clough's work, while the individual psychological
mechanisms available to each of the children were
essential in mediating the relationship between their
social experiences in home and in hospital, the whole
process was quite clearly socially situated.
    It is clear from the work surveyed and presented by
Clarke and Clarke (1976) that any notion of a simple
separation model with a biological base is insufficiently
sophisticated. The chapter by Rutter in that work draws
attention to this in relation to separation in hospital.
Particularly interesting is the finding that those children
who appear, over a long period of time, to suffer from a
stay in hospital are those children who are repeatedly
admitted to hospital and who are more likely to come from
disadvantaged homes.
    Another impediment to the recognition of the importance
of the variables to which we wish to draw attention is the
disease-cure model upon which modern medicine is based.
This point is also made by George Brown (1973) with regard
to mental hospitals. It is the business of medicine to
identify disease and to ameliorate or cure it. Ultimately
the purpose of this is that suffering shall be reduced,
but attention is directed to the disease rather than to
the suffering or the person who is suffering. The
concentration on disease seems to have the effect of
distracting attention from what cannot be defined as

disease, and therefore (unintentionally no doubt), to distract attention from, or to refuse to accept the evidence of, suffering which cannot be put down to an identifiable disease entity. Much of the evidence we have collected relates to suffering but not to suffering associated with disease entities.

The point made by Ruth Jacobs, about the failure to recognise or treat pain which is not physical pain, perhaps brings this out most strongly. She and Pill found that in the orthopaedic ward distress expressed post-operatively and therefore taken to be related to physical pain commanded respect and attention from the nursing staff. Distress expressed for other reasons did not command the same respect or attention and was more likely than post-operative distress to be ignored or dealt with impatiently. Their work and that of Cleary and Hall also gives the impression that staff were at a loss to know how to handle distress of psycho-social as opposed to physical origin. Jacobs pushes the point further, suggesting that the whole area of emotions is handled by denial: that rather than being treated, suffering which is of emotional origin is denied. Miller and Gwynne (1972) in their study of the incurably ill also eloquently show the distress caused by a failure to recognise the emotions patients are experiencing.

The problem of suffering

Our central concern is that unnecessary suffering should not be caused to children in the course of treating an ailment. Given this, it is important to remember, as Parsons (1951) has pointed out, that in our acceptance of medical practice we have accorded doctors the right to inflict pain. Our concern, therefore, has to be to see that doctors, nurses or other health workers do not inflict pain unnecessarily; we believe our skills as social scientists make it possible for us to point out the unintended suffering inflicted, suffering which is unrecognised and which may perhaps be unnecessary or avoidable. Our claim as sociologists and psychologists is to be able to observe and analyse such sufferings in dimensions where doctors and nurses are unsighted by virtue of their training. Their gaze is directed to the mysteries of physiology and anatomy, where their skills to see below the level of the obvious and commonsensical are today highly developed (Foucault, 1973). As social scientists our gaze has been trained to look at the workings of the mind and of society: what we deal with

are common sense and everyday concerns of all people as
social beings. It is our business to look below the
surface of the commonsensical and see the deeper
implications.

Perhaps some of us, as scientists, are embarrassed
to speak of suffering and unhappiness and feel that our
criteria should be objective and that we must justify
what we do in a utilitarian manner, showing, for example,
that expenditure on children now will avoid expenditure
on mental illness later. There is indeed something in
such arguments, but the approach has its pitfalls. It is
similar to that described by Macintyre (1977) for old age
during the 1950s and early 1960s when it was hoped that
active medical intervention aimed at rehabilitation of the
elderly and their return to their localities would result
at one and the same time in a reduction of individual
suffering among the elderly and reduced charges upon
society at large for the maintenance of the elderly.
Macintyre shows that there is a conflict between those two
aims such that both are unlikely to be equally well
achieved. So with children it is perhaps better to address
ourselves more directly to the reduction of suffering:
surely not a misplaced attention in a service whose very
aim it is to do just that.

It is sometimes argued that in matters of life and
death it is permissible that any and all procedures should
be undergone to save life and that in these circumstances
the finer considerations of feeling must be ignored. This
is part of the argument referred to earlier which treats
'welfare' as separate from 'real therapy'. Two questions
consequently arise: one is the point already made that
all the hazards of treatment processes should routinely be
taken into account and these include psycho-social hazards;
the second is that it becomes increasingly obvious that
life-saving at all costs, with the increased power of
contemporary medicine to keep people alive, if not to
cure them, is no longer an unproblematic goal. This last
point raises problems outside the scope of our present
work. In any case little of the daily routine of most
hospitals involves life-and-death situations.

There is a problem about unhappiness and suffering.
It can be argued with some reason that it is not the
business of doctors to treat unhappiness, that some
unhappiness is part of life; and here the whole argument
about the use and abuse of the increasing array of
psychotropic drugs is, of course, involved. We do not
wish to address these problems here. What we wish to
argue is that doctors, nurses and other health-care
professionals should come to understand   suffering which

is not caused by known disease entities may nevertheless
be systematically studied;   that a good deal of suffering
is caused to children by the very nature of the social
arrangements for treatment;   furthermore that the illness
and the treatment themselves may lead to suffering in
children which varies systematically from child to child.

In our view the model of medicine by which doctors work
has to be modified to take account of the kind of material
we have to offer. It is also up to us as social
scientists to try and present our material in such a way
that it can be usable. *First, however, it must be seen
to be acceptable.*

The acceptability and nature of social-science research

The present research was designed to throw light on some
dimensions of the treatment of children which fall outside
those areas dealt with systematically and scientifically
by contemporary medicine. The researches have attempted
to look in a sustained manner at areas which are generally
left to common sense and everyday knowledge: everyone
'knows' that children will be upset by going to hospital
but this is not something to worry about, it is part of
life, of growing up, of surviving. The research
inevitably, therefore, questions some of the taken-for-
granted assumptions upon which medicine is based and
hospitals are run. In this sense the research started
from a particular stance, as indeed must all research.
Within this stance it has attempted to be fair and
objective in its study.

Some who have read these accounts may have felt that
they are biased against doctors or nurses or hospitals.
This was not the intention: the intention was simply to
add a further dimension to the understanding of illness
and treatment in children. In so far as the findings are
critical of aspects of present practice, practitioners may
feel attacked, but the criticisms are of the practices of
a generation rather than of the performances of individuals
who, within the confines of contemporary medical understanding, provide good and helpful service. What we are
trying to do is address ourselves to an entire system of
knowledge and to suggest how it might be modified in the
better interests of the patients. Our findings call for
radical reappraisal and not the simple addition of new
techniques. In saying this we suggest that previous psycho-
social findings have been looked at as if they were mere
technique, resulting in the addition of a few new
practices, instead of being considered for their implications

for the social organisation of medicine and the nature of
medical knowledge. The reforms have therefore lost a good
deal of their force in practice.

Doctors constantly have to make decisions under pressure
and in the face of many unknowns, but at the same time in
highly repetitive and routine situations. They therefore
tend to work by certain rules of thumb. 'Children between
2 and 4 are vulnerable to separation in hospital' has
become one such. Where the paediatrician might extend this
rule to include children of other ages, it also becomes a
rule enforced by nurses and others and may be enshrined in
hospital regulations in some form. Thus a proposition
which starts as an indication that certain age groups are
more vulnerable than others to a stay in hospital can turn
into a hospital rule that those under 5, but no others,
can be visited freely. In this way a research finding is
assimilated to an ongoing set of values, attitudes and
relationships without the complex body of knowledge from
which it derived being in any way assimilated. To be fair
to the health-care professionals in this case, the
scientific message was fairly simple and rather narrow -
so much so that, as has been mentioned, the whole Bowlby
hypothesis is now coming under fire (Clarke and Clarke,
1976). Let us hope that this will not have the consequence
simply of increasing scepticism about the importance of the
psycho-social variables. The reasons for the criticisms
are indeed of a piece with our research findings. The
separation hypothesis is too simple and too generalised.
Our findings have taken us, as the previous chapters have
shown, well beyond separation as a cause of the unnecessary
and unintended suffering which child patients may find
themselves enduring.

The Court report itself (DHSS, 1976b) provides an example
of the partial assimilation of new learning. In the body
of that report a great deal of attention is paid to the
importance of social variables in illness, suffering and
treatment. There is not, however, a commensurate understanding demonstrated of the ways in which the organisation
of the hospital, of the health-care system and the imperatives of professionalism can themselves lead to unintended
suffering. Perhaps as a consequence, the implications of
a social understanding are not carried through to the
recommendations, either in terms of relationships with
parents, for which no structured arrangements are proposed,
or in terms of training implications. The education courses
suggested contain nothing on the sociology of health care
at all.

A new theoretical and philosophical approach to
treatment needed

What the researches have taught us is that additions must
be made to the body of knowledge used in modern medical
practice if unintended suffering is to be avoided.
Occasionally our findings emerge in easily grasped rules
of thumb;   more often they point to a need for a new
theoretical and philosophical approach on the part of
health-service workers and parents.   As such the findings
need discussion and assimilation before they can be
implemented, for the details have to be worked out for each
set of circumstances.

The first implication of our work, therefore, is that
health-care professionals should re-think the implications
of their work with children.   This re-thinking involves
the use of new concepts and has to proceed in two areas:
(i) the understanding of the child in relation to illness
and treatment and (ii) the understanding of the hospital
organisation.

UNDERSTANDING THE CHILD IN RELATION TO ILLNESS AND TREATMENT:
CATEGORISATION BY DISEASE INSUFFICIENT AS AN INDICATOR OF
SUFFERING

First it must be understood that the categorisation of
children by their diseases may not relate to the impact
(upon them as persons)of the disease and its treatment.
It is a matter of common observation that some children
admitted for the same illness and undergoing the same
treatment may suffer more than others.   These variations,
we have shown, can be systematically studied and explained.
The variations have to do with the social background of the
children, the kind of families they come from and the ways
in which they have learned to behave at home.

The initial pilot study suggested that children differed
systematically in their response to a short stay in hospital.
Thus Dearden (Stacey et al., 1970) suggested that the
vulnerable children tended to be only children or youngest
children in the family, to have a very bland or very anxious
mother and to have had less experience of meeting others.
Using quite different techniques, as he reports in chapter
2, Brown has supported the general tendency of these
findings except that he has found that only children tend
to be *less*, not more, distressed in hospital, although
youngest children tend to be more withdrawn.   What Brown
has shown is that the child's response in hospital varies
systematically with the characteristics of that child and

her/his family at home (Table 2.2). Those children who
were reported to score high on proximity - that is children
who, when at home, spent a lot of the time in the house,
in close proximity to other people and watched television
a lot - tended to score high for distress in hospital,
although they tended to be very mobile there. The child
likely to be distressed in hospital was also likely to be
one who did not initiate much at home, that is, was likely
to be controlled by others in the home situation and to
have less control (than high initiators) of what he/she
did, who he/she did it with, when and for how long.
Similarly the child who is withdrawn in hospital tends to
be a low initiator at home. The child who is not mobile
about the ward in hospital comes from a low-proximity family
and is a low initiator. Furthermore, there are relationships between the attitude of the mother and the child's
response in hospital: mothers who are highly accepting of
hospital authority tend to have children who are highly
distressed in hospital; mothers who express general
anxiety about their children tend to have children who are
not mobile in the hospital ward; mothers who are anxious
about hospital for themselves tend to have children who
are withdrawn when in hospital (Table 2.7). It is likely
that these maternal attitudes are linked with different
sorts of families as social environments.

The importance of family background

It is not only in terms of correlations between reported
child-rearing practices and behaviour at home that systematic
relationships are found between children from different
social situations and response in hospital. Brown also
studied the concept of proximity under controlled conditions.
Here he showed that high visual contact between mother and
child in the experimental situation is positively related
to proximity in the family situation and to mothers who
accept hospital authority and who were anxious about their
child, all factors which have been shown to relate to the
child's hospital response. Having also drawn in findings
from the Bene-Anthony family-relationship test, Brown was
able to conclude that the child vulnerable to short stay
in hospital was one who, more than others, limited her/his
view to family members and was highly ambivalent about
siblings. Brown is able to predict therefore that severe
problems will arise for a child in hospital, compared with
others who are undergoing the same illness and treatment
problems, when separation occurs in a family context which
emphasises the need for family members to be physically

close to each other and where there is ambivalence about
siblings.   The child who is particularly likely to exhibit
distress in hospital may be identified through the dynamics
of the family and the child's social position in the
family.

There is no doubt that while this last generalisation
is true, the details of Barrie Brown's findings are unlikely
to be the last word upon this complex subject: an understanding which began with separation and its importance
has already been both narrowed and widened, narrowed in
that separation may not have all the consequences claimed
for it, widened in that many other psycho-social variables
are now seen to be relevant to the suffering that illness
and treatment may involve for the child.   It is not
surprising that complete understanding has yet to be
reached.   Furthermore, one cannot rest too many conclusions
upon what was a limited study of a particular category of
children in a short-stay situation.   Further research is
needed to validate present findings and to advance the
limited understanding that has been achieved.

The meaning of illness and treatment to patients

Clough's data also provide evidence that the disease
category of the patient is likely to explain the meaning
of illness and treatment for her/him only in a very partial
manner.   As his chapter recounts, the meaning of illness
and treatment for girls of 9-16 years of age undergoing
orthopaedic treatment varied systematically in psycho-
social ways.   Clough shows the importance of the means-end
relationship as the patient perceives it.   He assumes that
when the patient defines herself as ill and at the same
time evaluates her treatment favourably in functional
and/or emotional terms, she should be positively motivated,
on both accounts, to accept hospital treatment.   Conversely,
if she does not define herself as ill, and also regards
medical treatment unfavourably, she should be negatively
motivated to reject hospital treatment.   A conceptual
conflict may arise when the patient defines herself as ill
and yet disvalues her treatment as disfunctional or
emotionally stressful: here she has simultaneous tendencies
to accept *and* reject treatment.   Where a patient defines
herself as not ill and her treatment as functional and
not stressful, this is a definition of perceived recovery,
satisfaction, or motivational relief (Figure 3.4).   These
different interpretations of events suggest potentially
different behavioural outcomes.   Clough distinguishes
theoretically four resultant groups which, upon analysis

of his data, he finds also exist in practice (Figure 3.5):

(i) A group of girls who perceive themselves as ill and accept treatment, who can therefore be expected to exhibit low anxiety and high co-operativeness and compliance.

(ii) A group of girls who perceive themselves as ill and yet reject treatment, who can therefore be expected to rate high on anxiety because of high motivational conflict but nevertheless to be compliant.

(iii) A group of girls who do not perceive themselves as ill and reject treatment, who therefore are opposed to the treatment offered or imposed and may be expected to be relatively non-compliant and unco-operative.

(iv) A group of girls who do not perceive themselves as ill but do accept treatment, who can therefore be expected to have a low motivation for treatment but low conflict and general satisfaction since they perceive themselves as recovered or recovering.

These and other analyses which Clough undertook suggest that 'there is consistent and striking evidence that disorders of behaviour are related to disorders of meaning described in terms of conceptual conflict, incongruity and dissonance'. Emotional stability and compliance are related to cognitive consistency and meaningfulness. The best predictor of a girl's hospital behaviour was her definition of her hospital situation.

Care must be taken in the interpretation of these findings, for it does not follow that non-compliant behaviour is necessarily wrong. As Stimson has shown, disobeying doctor's orders may sometimes be the only rational course of action (Stimson, 1974). Where non-compliance derives from misunderstanding about the nature and meaning of treatment the disobedience may be misplaced. On the other hand, a perception that the treatment is disfunctional may be well founded.

Older children and separation

As we have seen, Brown has shown that separation alone is not sufficient to account for a child's behaviour in hospital. Indeed from his work and that of others, it is also clear that some children ride the experience of going to hospital much better than others. Some of Brown's children were reported improved on some dimensions, and Douglas (1975) also reports that some pre-school children appear to benefit by a hospital stay. At the same time Clough's evidence suggests that separation stress is not confined to pre-school children. His female patients saw their world as divided into four areas: home life;

ward life; medical treatment; and illness. Each of these
was structured in terms of three independent dimensions of
meaning: Did it work? (functional evaluation); Was it
predictable? (predictability); Did it hurt? (stressfulness)
(Figure 3.2). The girls tended to see home life as
functional, predictable and not stressful; ward life was
not seen as stressful but as unpredictable and disfunctional;
medical treatment was seen as functional but stressful and
unpredictable; whereas illness was seen as predictable but
disfunctional and stressful. As Clough says, it is clear
that the girls were able to construct realistic ambivalent
conceptions, for example of medical treatment, in a way
that younger children would not be able to do. At the
same time the contrast they see between ward life and home
life suggests that even at this age separation and social
discontinuity are experienced. Clough found that this
discrepancy between a valued home life and a disvalued
ward life, which the girls perceived, was significantly
associated with reported anxiety behaviour independent of
illness-treatment conceptions. It would seem logical
therefore that we should be aware of distress arising from
separation not just in the pre-school child but in
children of all ages and indeed probably also in adults.
At the same time Clough shows that, for teenage girls at
least, sociability in the ward increases with familiarity
with the group setting, that is with length of stay, and
appears to be an independent function unrelated to illness-
treatment perceptions and their emotional concomitants
(Figure 3.3).

One of the interesting features of Clough's work is
that he shows something of the way in which broad sociological variables work their way through to the behaviour
of the girls in the ward. His path analysis suggests that
background variables like prior illness and hospitalisation and family status do not predict patient behaviour
directly but are mediated by the personal definitions which
the patients put upon their situation. He considers that
the background variables act to modify the patients'
perceptions and in this way indirectly influence their
behaviour. Similarly, the belief systems with which
patients identify appropriate ends and means of hospitalisation are themselves socially determined and subject to
cultural variation.

The evidence summarised above should be sufficient to
justify the first re-thinking which is here asked for,
namely that categorisation by disease is insufficient as
an indicator of the suffering that a patient may be
experiencing. It should also be sufficient to support the
second re-thinking that we are asking for: namely, that

recognition should be given to the complexity of the
subject. Psycho-social suffering may arise from a wide
variety of causes, but it can be identified and understood
in systematic ways. It will take much patient work to
unravel the mechanisms by which the effects of illness and
treatment emerge in suffering in children, and the
circumstances in which stress situations can be well
sustained. Continued and careful work will be necessary
before any full understanding can be reached. The first
step is that there should be an awareness of the complexity
and therefore that there should be sensitivity in practice.

THE HOSPITAL ORGANISATION:
NEED TO MODIFY HOSPITAL INSULARITY

Earlier it was pointed out that a major implication of our
work is that health-care professionals must think of their
work in new ways if they are to avoid unnecessary suffering
to child patients. This re-thinking was divided into two
parts: (i) an understanding of the child in relation to
health and illness and (ii) an understanding of the hospital
as a social organisation. Because of the existence of the
hospital as the locus of treatment and also because what
is treated there is a disease and not a person, the care
of the child tends to be fragmented; but the child is a
whole person and the way she/he is treated in hospital, or
indeed that she/he is treated in hospital at all, is a
part of her/his total life. Pill has shown that in understanding what illness and treatment mean to a child, and
also to some extent the child's family, the notion of
health and treatment careers can be helpful. Obviously,
in one sense an approach of this kind is common in medical
practice in so far as the medical history is taken into
account in coming to a decision about diagnosis and
treatment. The proposal here is that account should also
be taken, as a matter of routine, of the social aspects
of the child's history since these may be determinant in
treatment and outcome. In practice this cannot be done
without modifying the insularity of the hospital.

Hospital as one episode in child's health and treatment
career

Instead of seeing children as being in hospital for a
specific condition, Pill sees them as being there because
they have a particular health career, in which the pattern
of contact with health agencies is most important.

Children who have similar impairment and a similar
prognosis (that is, the same health status and whose
potential has therefore been defined as similar) may
follow quite different treatment paths. Therefore,
although they start out with the same life-chances, they
may well experience quite different lives. These
differences may emerge because of contact with various
health professionals who define the action to be taken
differently; for example, of two similar cases one may
be treated at outpatients, another admitted. Pill found,
however, that children from different social backgrounds
but with the same health status are apt to follow different
health and treatment careers. This may occur because of
the parents' lack of skill in convincing the doctor that
they are able to carry out the treatment and care themselves,
or alternatively, that there is a case for their child to
be admitted. Pill shows that the long-stay patients (that
is, those who have been in hospital for more than four
months) are a heterogeneous category, and illuminates their
variety by using the concept of career. She shows that
while most can be presumed to have been admitted to hospital
for medical reasons, some are undoubtedly there for social
reasons, because their families cannot cope with their
impairment. This is not a matter merely, or even necessarily,
of economic circumstance. Nor is it a matter for moral
opprobrium. It may arise from inadequate housing, because
the parent has no spouse or because of a lack of support
in a social and emotional sense among the collectivity of
family members. These factors are added to the doctor's
definition of parental competence already mentioned.
Looking at a child's health career leads the observer to
see the decision to admit or discharge as part of an on-
going interaction process involving the doctors, the child
and the family. One factor in this is the parents'
definition of the situation, which involves their assessment of the child's health status and the impact of that
on the life of the family and their attitude to it at
that time. Many of these factors are of course recognised
by practitioners dealing with children but they seem to be
seen as peripheral to the decisions concerned with diagnosis
and treatment rather than as integral to them. Pill's
evidence suggests that although unrecognised in any
systematic way these factors are in fact integral to the
decisions taken. The proposal here is that their essential
role in therapy should be recognised.
    The point is that children may get differential
treatment not only because their initial health status
leads to variations in their life-chances but because of
social variations also. A conscious effort therefore has

to be made to ensure that children from more socially
disadvantaged homes whose health status is impaired are
not doubly disadvantaged by spending their lives in a
deprived environment. This can come about either because
there is inadequate provision for the support of families
or because residential accommodation alternative to the
hospital is not available for handicapped children. Pill
shows that, not only do hospital staff tend to see the
child's career solely in terms of that part of it which
involves their hospital stay, but also that administrative
categories are too static to reveal a picture of the
processes which are affecting the child. Thus administrative divisions into short-stay and long-stay patients
ignore completely the dynamic of the repeat admission.
Increasingly children are discharged after a relatively
short stay to be readmitted after a while for further
treatment. This is a category to which more attention
should be paid. The emotional and social stresses imposed
by repeat admissions upon the child and her/his family are
little understood. Rutter has recently reported (Clarke
and Clarke, 1976) that repeated hospital admissions are
significantly associated with later psychiatric disturbance
where the first admission occurred before the age of 5
years but this was most likely to occur in children who
came from homes which were psycho-socially disadvantaged.

Discontinuity between hospital and home

It is clear that in the case of repeated admissions the
way in which links between the home and the hospital are
forged is of the utmost importance. Yet there is mounting
evidence that there are major discontinuities experienced
both by the child and the child's family in the continuity
of care between the home and the hospital. Elsewhere,
Pill and Jacobs (1974) report that parents did not receive
adequate help with aids for orthopaedic patients discharged
from hospital, a matter which occasioned considerable
distress and difficulty. Harrisson (1974), working
independently in another part of the country, arrived at
the same conclusion. In addition, Clough (1975) found
that no attention was paid to the difficulties parents
might have in maintaining contact with their children
admitted to hospital for scoliosis treatment. The choice
of hospital for admission appeared not to be made on
rational medical grounds, as being that hospital which
had a treatment method most suited to the particular case,
nor on grounds of social convenience, as being the most
accessible. Referral appeared to be rigidly routine in

most cases.   Clough argues reasonably that where the
medical success of the outcomes of various treatments is
not clearly established, social and emotional factors
should also be taken into account.   These factors should
include the preferences of the parents or the child for
one treatment or another, and the cost and difficulty of
getting to the hospital for the parents, particularly in
cases where treatment is going to be prolonged.   The
evidence collected by the Welsh Hospital Board (1972),
also suggests that when one looks at the matter from the
point of view of the parents and children, there are great
discontinuities in the provision of health care between
home and hospital.   Factors of great importance to the
child and family in terms of successful outcome are quite
ignored by those who only have a hospital orientation.
Sociologically one would expect that among those situated
in hospitals such a perspective would inevitably tend to
develop.   It is for this reason that the routine application of a concept like health career is important to
counteract this tendency.

The hospital as a social organisation, a discontinuous
environment

This discussion of health and treatment careers has already
drawn attention to one aspect of the hospital as a social
organisation in its consequences for therapy: this is
the facet of the hospital as a discrete locus which has
the consequences of introducing sequential discontinuity
into the child's therapy.   In addition we have drawn
attention in this volume to various features of the
hospital as a social organisation, which features may
have unfortunate unintended consequences for child patients.
Our argument here is that rather than conceiving of the
hospital as a rational organisation designed to facilitate
treatment with the greatest possible efficiency, the
hospital in addition is, and should be conceived as, a
social organisation which is full of discontinuities for
the child patient, which fragments the child and her/his
care, which is resistant to change, and where information
control is used to maintain the status quo.   At the same
time any hospital as an on-going concern is a social
organisation which is the result of the problem-solving
activities of those who are within it, especially of
those who work there, and which is therefore subject to
modification.   We therefore see our invitation to re-think
the hospital as a prelude to some reorganisation in
the interests of better therapy.

A child coming into hospital has already suffered discontinuity of social relationships but the social relationships within the hospital are themselves characterised by discontinuities. At home the child has had contact with a limited number of people and therefore has experienced a limited range of variation and inconsistency in social contacts and, furthermore, has become familiar with that range. The younger the child the more true that is likely to be. In hospital the child meets very many people, all initially strangers. Furthermore, as Hall shows, these people are not consistent among themselves in their approach to children. There was, for example, no clear policy on how to deal with disruptive children and depending on which nurse was on duty and handling the child, so the child might be treated differently: a source of discontinuity.

Patient assignment desirable

Other discontinuities are a function of the formal work organisation, as, for example, the task-based allocation of work to nurses, so graphically described by Cleary in chapter 5. She showed how the children are deprived of understanding and comfort because the style of work allocation prevents the nurses' attention being drawn to the individual needs of children and prevents the staff seeing the child as a whole person. Where nurses' work is allocated by task and not by patient, the care of any one patient is inevitably fragmented. Given the rapid turnover of patients in modern wards and the personnel changes involved in the shift system, nurses are unlikely to come to know children as whole persons. Not only this, but the focus of the nurses' work is certain physical and definable jobs which must be done. This may not even be the most appropriate way of ensuring a child gets the right physical treatment, for which some continuity of care is essential. Certainly, as Jacobs points out, it prevents attachments developing and, as she shows, and as Cleary emphasises, features of the ward organisation can have the effects of creating an emotionally deprived environment for the child. Our conclusion from these findings is that patient assignment rather than task assignment would reduce the discontinuities suffered by the child in hospital. We note that this is also strongly advocated by the Expert Group on Play for Children in Hospital (DHSS, 1976a). It has been suggested by various people over the years but there appears to be resistance to the implementation of the proposal. We think this

derives from the way in which the nursing task is conceived
and feel that the re-thinking of therapy which we are
asking for is probably necessary before nurses will see
the point of reorganising their whole manner of working.

Denial of emotions reinforced by hospital organisation

Jacobs has also drawn attention to the fragmentation of
care and is probably right when she argues by implication
that this fragmentation can only be overcome if the
emotions which the staff experience in nursing children
and the emotions which the children experience are recognised
and mechanisms devised for dealing with them. At present,
as she argues, the practices and procedures of the hospital
sustain a system in which emotions are denied. The
fragmentation of nursing care involved in task assignment
is one of these procedures. As Parsons (1951) has pointed
out the ideal-typical model of the doctor-patient relationship (and this applies to all relationships between
health-care professionals and their clients) is affect-
free. Yet we have to recognise that when a ward is run
in a way which prevents the expression of emotions and
indeed denies them, it does not produce for the patient
an emotionally or morally neutral environment. It produces
an environment which may appear to the patient at best as
cold and unsupportive and at worst actually hostile,
although it may also be an environment in which some find
it easier to survive. Clough's adolescent girls found the
ward was disfunctional and unpredictable. The discontinuities and the fragmentation of care would seem to be
part of the explanation for this.

Jacobs also suggests that the hierarchical structure of
the hospital organisation was itself a mechanism which
supported the fragmentation and the denial of emotions.
The social and the emotional life of the staff was circumscribed while they were in the hospital, and many of
them lived there. Higher echelons lived much of their
life away from the hospital, but those who came most into
contact with the children were the most junior and least-
trained staff, and it was they who were most restrained.
The rigid hierarchical system confined the free expression
of emotions to equals. Those with more experience who
might have been able to help younger staff over difficult
feelings never learned what those feelings were. Jacobs
observed no ways in which suffering experienced by staff
was recognised or handled. Hall reports that dealing
with dying children was felt by nurses in his ward to be
the most difficult thing they had to do, and staff in

Jacobs' ward found difficulty when they were assigned to
nurse an irrevocably and badly brain-damaged child who
had been battered, or children suffering from progressive
degenerative disease for whom little could be done.
Recognition was accorded to their difficulties only by
removing them from the assignment: the difficulties
were not overtly recognised or worked through. It was
not part of their training to be taught to understand
emotions.

This, as we have argued above, is part of the modern
medical model for dealing with emotions, as Parsons has
shown. What we are arguing now is that the entire social
structure of the hospital tends to reinforce this model
in which the symptoms are detached from the person manifesting them and in which staff relate to the children
less as persons and more as objects with certain physiological needs which are to be met through certain technical
procedures. When these needs were low the children
received little attention.

There is no doubt that this approach and the discipline
which goes with it is one way of coping with the complex
problems which medical treatment imposes upon practitioner
and patient alike. Our point is that it is part of a
structure of belief and behaviour which may have unfortunate consequences for some children. It may, of
course, produce an environment in which some children get
on better than they do at home. This may be one of the
explanations for the finding that some children improve
after a stay in hospital and certainly has to be part of
the explanation of why some children sustain hospital so
much better than others.

The hospital as a negotiated order

Our work has shown that the hospital is not only a
formally organised social system but is also a social
order established as a result of negotiations among all
the participants. There is within that organisation a
tendency for a variety of mechanisms to be used which have
the effect of maintaining the status quo, maintaining
such power and privilege as the participants may have
been able to achieve. Thus Jacobs shows how information
was withheld from parents and how their access to the ward
was restricted. This had the effect of reducing the threat
to the social order of the ward, which, as outsiders, they
represented. Hall (1977) shows how the playleader was
accorded a place lower than that of the nursing staff by
the withholding of information from her. She was inclined

initially to make mistakes because she had not been given
information about the children: the mistakes were held
against her. By withholding information power was
retained and a relatively lowly place ensured for her.
Information control is also a way of maintaining the
status quo in the relationship between staff and patients.
The scoliosis patients and their parents were not told
about the pathological consequences of the girl's condition,
which reduced their treatment motivation (Clough, 1975);
nor were thay told about the widely varying treatments
available for scoliosis, nor was the appropriateness of one
treatment rather than another for their particular case
discussed with them. Parents in all cases were given
minimum information about when their child would be called
to hospital, what would happen there or when she might be
discharged. The survey for the Welsh Hospital Board
showed that the more planned the admission the less
information the parents had (Stacey and Earthrowl, 1973).
It is a common observation that surveys which otherwise
show high satisfaction rates show high incidences of
dissatisfaction about the information made available to
the patient (e.g. Cartwright, 1964). We see this retention
as a way of reducing the uncertainty for the professionals
concerned. It increases uncertainty for the patient or
lower professional (e.g. Waitzkin and Stoeckle, 1972;
Waitzkin and Stoeckle, 1976). As such it is likely to
increase feelings of meaningless and powerlessness
experienced by those kept in ignorance.

Reasons for resistance to change in hospitals

Hospitals, like other social organisations, are likely
to be resistant to change unless the changes proposed are
in the interests of participants who are in a position to
achieve their ends. Where the changes are likely to
upset the interests of participants, they are likely to
be resisted. For all those in the ward there are uncertainties, as Hall argues above, perhaps greatest for
the children and their parents but by no means absent for
the staff, who are faced not only with negotiations with
other staff of various occupations and professions but
also with a not-altogether-predictable array of children
with ailments and treatments which may not take a typical
course. Any innovation in the ward increases the number
of problems to be solved, which may of itself be a reason
for resistance to the innovation. When the innovation
runs counter to traditional values, as occurred in the
case of the playleader, the problems are multiplied. The

presence of the playleader undoubtedly threatened the
work of the cleaners; the cleaners were able to invoke
the universal hospital values of cleanliness and tidiness
as being essential for therapy and to gain the support of
the nurses in this. The nurses were happy to have the
support of the playleader in looking after the children
but did not want their status in the ward undermined.
The resolution for the time being of the conflict between
the activities and the values of the playleader and the
activities of the nurses and cleaners was to isolate the
playleader both socially and spatially, confining her
activities as far as possible to the playroom. It was
implicitly understood that the playleader would look after
the relatively well children in the playroom, leaving the
nurses freer to concentrate their professional attention
on the sick children in the ward.

Hall also found that the hierarchical division in the
hospital structure had an effect in impeding innovation.
The consultants were supportive of the work that the playleaders were doing but were not present in the ward often
or long enough for their potential support for the
innovation to be developed. In the earlier studies Pill
(Stacey et al., 1970) showed how the innovation of
permitting parents unrestricted visiting was effectively
blocked by nurses at the ward level because it was upsetting
to their work situation and there was nobody else present
in the wards to ensure that the policy was operated.

The future for play in hospital

Hall and Cleary show, and Hall's findings in chapter 7
underline, that attempts to ameliorate the circumstances
of children in hospital run counter to the basic conceptions of hospital staff as to what hospital should be
about and what the priorities established there should be.
Play is not seen as integral to treatment but as peripheral
to it. In this context the response to the report of the
Expert Group on play in hospital (DHSS, 1976a) is interesting.
That group recommended that special playworkers should be
employed in the ratio of 1 to every 8 or 10 children, that
is, at least 10 playworkers for a large district general
hospital; that they should be independent of nursing staff
and of occupational therapists and that they should have
their own Whitley grading. The Expert Group made this
recommendation because they felt 'that the nature of the
work involved and the demands for the foreseeable future
on nursing staff make it unrealistic to expect nurses
employed as such to take total responsibility for developing

play in the wards' (para. 3.7). Also local education authorities' recently expanded commitments in the fields of nursery education and mental handicap may mean that many will be unable to undertake further responsibility in hospitals, or at least not to the level required to obviate special provision for play by Area Health Authorities (para. 4.4).

The DHSS has rejected this advice and suggested instead that play should become part of nurses' work with children, that nurses should be given some special training to this end and that a senior nurse should be specially designated to encourage play. Economy grounds are given for this conclusion but one cannot help feeling that the DHSS may not have been uninfluenced by representatives from the nursing profession who may have felt their position in relation to child patients threatened by the proposal of a new profession of playworkers.

The DHSS has accepted the therapeutic advantages of encouraging play among children in hospital. It has adopted a solution which the Expert Group had concluded would not result in sufficient encouragement of play. The Expert Group's evidence, which was supported by the fate of the nursery nurses employed under HM(61) 68 ('Employment of Nursery Nurses in Hospital') who tended to be absorbed into general nursing duties, is also supported by the evidence from all our studies. We note that the Court Report (DHSS, 1976b) regrets the DHSS decision, and doubts if there are adequate numbers of nurses to meet the need for play. Given economic constraints Court recommends an extended use of volunteers (para. 12.42).

It may be that if play is made a formal nursing task, a start can be made upon what is after all one of our major recommendations, namely that welfare be integrated with therapy. The training necessary to teach nurses to play with children, if carried out, will inevitably go some way towards our recommendation that nurses should be taught about the social, emotional and educational needs of the children in their care. Perhaps such a development will help to change the present rather narrow bias of the clinical model which has dominated nurse-training in the past. If so this would be entirely in line with what we have in mind in this volume. We remain unconvinced that this one element of a broader approach is likely to survive its encounters with the dominant values of the clinical model either in training or in practice. The intention is an interesting one, however, and constitutes a test of our findings. We would, therefore, propose that the developments which follow the recommendations of health

circular HC(76)5 'Play for Children in Hospital' be
carefully surveyed and attention paid to the amount of
success with which the recommendations are attended.
However successful the integration of play into the work
of nurses with children may be, there is one grave disadvantage in the proposal, a disadvantage which cannot be
overcome without a radical reorganisation of nursing as an
occupation. We have shown in this and other works that a
major source of discontinuities for the child in the ward
comes from the large number of different people to whom
the child has to relate during the course of her/his
hospital stay. We have shown, also, that the people with
whom the child comes most into contact are the least trained
- the pupils and the students. One of the great merits of
the playworker proposal was that it would provide continuity of contact for the child with trained personnel.
This the nurses cannot provide because of their shift
system and because of training on the job.

Importance of institutionalised links with world outside

It is interesting that the **Expert** Group proposed that the
playworkers should be responsible to the Area Health
Authority. In addition to being independent of the nursing
staff, which our research findings also led us to recommend,
it was our view that play people would be better employed
by local education authorities rather than by health
authorities. Education authorities already have considerable responsibilities in hospitals and so have experience
on which to build an on-going involvement. It was our
view that they should also accept responsibility for play
because we felt that the medical values are so dominant
throughout the health authority that the playworkers would
be strengthened by support from an independent outside
organisation. We have also been impressed in all our
hospital studies (not only those specifically concerned
with playleaders) by the tendencies of hospitals as
organisations to become closed. We think that this can
lead to an isolated environment and one which is more at
variance with the outside world than the needs of illness
and treatment really demand. This phenomenon increases
the discontinuities which the children may suffer. It is
our belief, therefore, that the more institutionalised
ties linking the hospital with the outside world the
better.

Parents as negotiators in the ward

The parents, of course, except for the few children
abandoned in long-stay care, constitute the strongest
institutionalised link between the child patients and the
outside world. In our studies we recorded the frequency
of parental visiting and something of the interactions
of parents with their children. While it was not a main
focus of our studies, we do have evidence of the role
parents played in on-going negotiations in the ward.

In the case of the orthopaedic hospital, the parents
were there in most cases for so relatively small an
amount of time that their impact could not be great and
our findings concentrated on the powerlessness of the
parents. Hall and Cleary's in-ward study shows how
parents have a different perspective on the ward interactions from the ward staff and perceived the children's
situation from a different viewpoint - often, we thought,
closer to the child's perception. Parents intervened to
help other children as well as their own and to interpret
their wishes in situations where the children's problems
were not understood by the staff, largely in consequence
of the fragmented nature of the care which we have already
discussed. Yet it is clear from our analyses that parents
are not brought fully into the ward life.

In our earlier studies Pill (Stacey et al., 1970)
pointed out the difficulties encountered by mothers and
staff in knowing how the role of mother-in-the-ward should
be played. This part has been played for many years now
but there is still uncertainty and diffidence (see also
Hales-Tooke, 1973). Emphasis has in the past been laid
upon what the hospital should do to help the parents play
their part and, undoubtedly, were hospitals conscientiously
to admit parents to full membership of their child's
caring team, the situation of parents in the ward would
be radically altered. Parents tend still to be treated
as outsiders and to be tolerated rather than integrated.
The Court Report (DHSS, 1976b) frequently argues against
this attitude and stresses the importance of a parent-
professional partnership in the interests of child health
(e.g. pp. 23, 54, 99, 179).

The result of our present researches and our understanding of the negotiated order of the ward suggests to
us that, given present ward regimes, there is a good deal
that parents can do to help create an environment in the
ward appropriate for their child and to create for themselves an active role. This may not always be easy for
parents to do because they are not expected to play an
active part in ward negotiations; indeed they tend to be

cast in a passive role by ward staff, a point well made by Webb (in Davis and Horobin, 1977).

Webb makes plain the relative powerlessness of the parents in the ward and our studies go some way to show why ward staff should wish parents to be compliant and non-interfering. At the same time Webb's study shows how parents, who have some understanding of the way the order of the ward is maintained and some conviction that they, as well as the experts, have a positive contribution to make towards their child's well-being, may intervene successfully on behalf of their children in the negotiations which sustain that order. Webb also noted that while the parents were very supportive to each other in private, sharing their anxieties about the way the children were being treated, parents did not support each other in attempts to change the treatment. Our studies support Webb's findings. Parents did not intervene much or collectively. Only a small minority of parents intervene: those perhaps who are supported by organisations such as the Association for the Welfare of Children in Hospital or the National Association for the Welfare of Children in Hospital. When such organisations encourage parents to enter negotiations on behalf of their children – for example, to be allowed to stay with them longer or to do more things for them – the organisations are encouraging parents to take a more active role. Such parents are often seen as 'difficult', because their requests may not be in the interests of the staff who are in a position to dominate the ward negotiations. At the same time our studies leave us in no doubt that the parents have a perspective of their child's situation and an understanding of it which, when taken into account in the care of the child, can decrease the discontinuities experienced by the children; ignoring this perspective is one way in which the discontinuities experienced by the children are increased.

Parents, as Webb shows, have a role to play in hospital, not only to maintain the parent-child bond during this stressful period for the children but also to give emotional support, to provide mental stimulation through play and to act as mediator on behalf of the child in relations with the staff. A parent can also, and it is part of the mediating role, act as a watch on the efficiency of the treatment, a function which in adult wards patients can do for themselves, and which patients do for each other when some of their number are very ill and dependent and unable to look out for themselves. Adolescent children are also able to help each other, as Clough has shown, but very small children cannot do this.

Webb also shows that only those mothers who were living in the ward really gained enough knowledge to play the mediating role effectively.

PRACTICAL RECOMMENDATIONS

We turn now to a consideration in detail of the practical recommendations which we wish to make. They fall under three main headings. The first is a programme of education and training designed to encourage the re-thinking which we feel is necessary; the second relates to organisational changes; and the third to further research which is needed.

1 EDUCATION AND TRAINING

1a Interdisciplinary discussion

We recommend that discussions should take place between social scientists and medical and other health-care practitioners about the relationship of findings such as ours to those which flow from more traditional medical approaches. This is essential if concerns about treatment processes and outcomes of the kind expressed here are not to be brushed aside as 'welfare' which can be ignored depending on the dictates of medical imperatives. Social scientists need to be in interaction with doctors, nurses and others about the implications of the findings for treatment in a variety of settings. More than a twenty-minute paper at a professional gathering or even a day or a half-day conference is needed. Something more like a continuing seminar is called for because it is not just a matter of assessing findings, it is a matter of working through concepts and of working through the implications of research findings in that light and in the practical circumstances in which practitioners find themselves. Parents and patients also need to be involved in discussions, for their viewpoint is valid in its own right and not just as mediated by social scientists.

1b Education

It is clear that the concepts used to understand the socio-logical and psychological aspects of treatment go well beyond those which are the common stock in trade of those employed in the health service. It is, therefore,

essential that all these practitioners become familiar
with them if research findings such as these are to be
understood in anything other than a common-sense way as
'mere opinion' (or even intelligent advice). A serious
approach to this must therefore be made at the level of
postgraduate or post-credential education. At this level
the proposal is an adjunct to the working seminar proposal
embedded in recommendation la above.

Increasingly, sociology and psychology are included in
medical and nursing education. This will clearly help.
Questions may still be asked as to whether enough is
included or at the right stage but if these courses are
simply seen as something aside from the mainstream of
medical education, the failure to assimilate psychological
and sociological approaches into the mainstream medical
model will continue. This means that the social sciences
should be seen as basic sciences and given an equal weight
with the natural sciences in medical education - they
should constitute half the work of the pre-clinical years,
knowledge of them should be tested as rigourously, and
their satisfactory completion should be a requirement for
proceeding as in the case of any of the traditional
sciences. Furthermore, the social sciences must continue
to be taught in the clinical years, so that the early
learning is constantly reinforced in practice. There is
a difficulty here of linking teaching about social interaction and social systems with teaching about individual
cases. Clinical teaching concentrates on the individual
case, at present on the disease entity. This can be
extended to include some social and psychological factors
but those sociological features of treatment which relate
to medical organisation must form a subject of study
separate from the clinical case. The hospital or the ward,
for example, must become a subject for applied study, but
this is to look far beyond the present organisation of
medicine. Within the present context perhaps the most
one can ask for is for continuing attention to be paid
to sociological and psychological facets in the clinical
years.

The success of including social-science components in
the education of doctors, nurses and others must, therefore,
depend partly on the success of seminars and of postgraduate education linked with more specific health and
treatment issues of the kind outlined in la above. This
is important because if those clinicians who are involved
in teaching have not come to understand the relevance of
the social-science component the teaching of the pre-
clinical years may very well be largely lost. If seminars
and postgraduate education are on-going and assimilation

of knowledge begins, practitioners will become supportive
of the knowledge which students are gaining and reinforce
it in practice.

2 ORGANISATIONAL CHANGES

2a The hospital as the locus of health care

As modern medicine has developed, the hospital has become
the central locus of health care. The origins of modern
hospitals are various - shelters for the sick poor,
segregation for the contagious or infectious, training
centres for medical students. During the nineteenth century
the clinical model came to dominate and the locus of
treatment has gradually been removed from the home to the
hospital over the past 150, and especially the past 75,
years (Abel-Smith, 1964; Foucault, 1967). The hospital
as a form of social organisation has therefore been
closely associated with that particular approach to disease
and illness which is characterised by modern clinical
medicine and the organisation of the hospital has been
dominated by the perceived medical needs of the practice
of such medicine. If, as we recommend, psychological and
sociological facets of illness and treatment are assimilated
to the traditional medical approach, it will be seen that
the form of the hospital will have to change. In particular,
the isolation of the hospital from the wider society must
be overcome. Some moves are already afoot to this end and
need encouraging and reinforcing.

(i) *The involvement of parents in the care of their
children in hospital*. This is a well-established and
long-standing policy which should be reinforced and
developed not only because of the hazards of the separation of the child from her/his mother but in order to
reduce to some extent the many discontinuities which the
child suffers. It is important as a part of a policy to
reduce the isolation of the hospital as a social
organisation.

(ii) *The involvement of school teachers, nursery
teachers and playworkers employed by the local education
authority in the hospital* is recommended, so that their
expertise and their standards and values shall have
expression there, thus reducing the isolation of the
hospital and increasing the continuity of practices and
procedures from the outside world.

(iii) *The access of siblings* may sometimes be most
important, especially for some of the vulnerable young
child patients.

(iv) For adolescents the *access of their peers* may be especially important.

(v) *The involvement of health visitors from the district in the hospital wards*. This is already done in some hospitals and helps to provide continuity of care between home and the hospital.

(vi) The employment of *foster grannies* now being developed in some hospitals should be encouraged.

(vii) *The involvement of consultants in clinics in localities outside the hospital*. This is already practised as far as some specialities are concerned. The network of orthopaedic outpatient clinics which runs from Oswestry throughout North Wales is a good and long-established example. The newer developments of community paediatricians may also be mentioned. The advantages of this kind of development were argued by the Welsh Hospital Board's working party (1972) for paediatricians but could well be applied to other specialities also. Health centres and the surgeries of group practices are foci where cases could be gathered together for the consultant to see. It would have the merit for the consultant of taking her/him from the hospital to other locales, have the merit for the general practitioner in bringing her/him closer to hospital procedure and practice, and afford an excellent teaching opportunity thus helping to maintain high standards of general practice.

We are pleased to note that the Court Report (DHSS, 1976b) recommends the attendance of consultant paediatricians at health centres and group practices (para. 7.33). However it is a matter of regret that the report nevertheless suggests the appointment of a separate category of community paediatricians in addition to the existing hospital-based consultant paediatricians and community physicians (child health).

(viii) *The development of paediatric home-nursing schemes*, whereby children are nursed at home according to the instructions of the relevant consultant but under the care of the general practitioner and attended by specially trained nurses. Ideally there should be some exchange of nurses working in hospital with those nursing children in their own homes, so that the same nurses should have a clear understanding of the characteristics and problems of each environment.

While the Court Report suggests the development of a child-nursing service to help nurse children in their own homes (op. cit., pp. 301-2) and advocates trained hospital staff to advise child-health visitors, the report does not go so far as to suggest that the same personnel should nurse both in hospital and at home.

(ix) *The reduction of admissions for observation by the increased collection of specimens* in the GP's surgery or at outpatients rather than admitting the child.

(x) *Attention should be paid by child-health teams to the continuity of care between hospital and home,* particularly after discharge, and to the analysis of treatment patterns using the concepts of health and treatment careers. In this connection particular attention should be paid to ensure that children from more socially disadvantaged homes are not doubly disadvantaged by spending their lives in a deprived environment.

(xi) The almost complete absence of medical social workers from the wards we studied means that we have no direct experience of their work. We note that the Working Party on Children in Hospital in Wales (WHB, 1972) advocates their greater use.

2b The organisation of the hospital

The recommendations in 2a above will themselves bring in their train changes in the organisation of the hospital, both because of the reorganisation of work patterns they would involve and because of the changed staff attitudes which would ensue. In addition certain specific modifications are suggested.

(i) *Children should always be nursed on the basis of patient assignment* rather than task assignment.

(ii) *The involvement of all staff concerned with child care in conferences* about the progress of the children, whether they are hospital staff or local authority staff.

(iii) *Clear arrangements to be made for information about the child's progress to be made available to parents and guardians.* Consultants or their nominees should be available to answer questions at clearly publicised times. The willingness of the ward sister to answer questions and where and how to find her should be made plainer to parents. An information kiosk in the hospital also has much to commend it, where general questions about facilities and where to go and what to do may be addressed.

(iv) *Nurses, especially those in training, should be specifically helped to understand the complex emotions which they experience in nursing sick and dying children* and to understand emotional problems of their child patients. Emotional support of the patient should be recognised as a technical nursing task.

(v) *Regular reviews of rules and procedures* undertaken with the question in mind: 'Do we do it this way because it is in our interests as staff and more

comfortable for us or do we do it this way because it is
in the child's best interest?'
   (vi) *Regular collection of the child's point of view*
should take place. Some paediatricians have found that
asking patients to write essays about being in hospital
can be most illuminating.
   (vii) *Regular collection of the views of patients'
parents* is also important and can be done at intervals by
the use of a standardised questionnaire, and would keep
all staff alert to the parents' point of view. This is
not, however, a substitute for parents' organisations which
can enter into negotiations with hospital staff about
conditions for the patients.

2c The role and responsibilities of parents

   (i) In our view *parents have an important contribution
to make* with regard to their child's welfare in hospital.
They constitute the major link for the child between the
hospital and the outside world. While, as we have just
suggested, the hospital has a responsibility to solicit
the parental view, parents also have a responsibility to
ensure that that view is put forward. This is, as we have
seen, difficult for parents to do because such behaviour
falls outside the ethos and expectations of staff in the
ward, outside assumptions about the active expert who
knows best, and the passive recipient of skilled care.
But there is a sense in which parents have a special skill
in relation to their own children, skills of knowledge and
understanding. Where parents are able to be present with
their children they can help reduce the discontinuities for
them by acting as supporter, mediator and stimulator
throughout the treatment process. In doing this they have
to create a role and enter into many and varied interactions
in the ward.
   (ii) We see, therefore, *an important role for organisations* like the Association for the Welfare of Children in
Hospital and the National Association for the Welfare of
Children in Hospital and other specialist groups concerned
with children: to support individual parents in the ward,
to provide them with a point of reference from which they
may be able to play an active rather than a passive parent
role; to provide parents with a source of knowledge and
information about the ways of hospitals, what services
are available, what normal practice is, what best practice
is, how to find one's way through the hierarchy; and last
but by no means least to put forward the parents' point
of view, collectively, to the health-care professionals
and the administrators.

(iii) At present such organisations have not enough members to provide a continuous presence in every hospital ward where children are nursed. Most parents will therefore have to be reliant upon their own resources in negotiations for their children. We would advise *parents to help each other* in the difficulties they encounter in wards and departments.

These proposals are not made in any sense of anatagonism towards the staff, but because of the importance of reducing discontinuities if the suffering of children is to be minimised.

(iv) In view of the importance of the parent to the sick child a *child-sickness benefit* should be payable to parents (either mother or father) to permit them to take time off work to be with their sick children.

2d The role of the general practitioner

It is clear that the GP plays an important part in a child's treatment career in hospital in so far as he/she acts as a gatekeeper to the hospital service and is responsible for the medical care of the child after discharge from hospital. GPs can clearly help initially by discussing with parents any alternative referral procedures that might be possible, by taking the psychological and social circumstances of the child and family into account when making referrals and by encouraging parents to play a supportive role towards their children in hospital. GPs have a particularly crucial role in the career and treatment of permanently impaired children whose future depends so much on how they are classified and where and in what manner they are treated. The importance of sending the specimen rather than the patient to hospital has already been mentioned in 2a (ix) above.

We are aware that GPs have problems in communication with hospitals and particularly in receiving sufficiently soon information about discharged patients. This is part of the hiatus between hospital and home to which we have referred. We feel that GPs should be supported in any attempts they make to get these communications improved and that GPs in their turn should support the efforts which we hope child-health teams will make to improve the continuity of care between home and hospital (see 2a (x) above).

3 FURTHER RESEARCH

(i) The research into the vulnerability of pre-school children to a short stay in hospital is the most advanced. This has reached the stage where an instrument for the detection of particularly vulnerable children before or at admission could be developed. High priority should be given to such research for, were it possible to detect vulnerability, either the admission could be postponed or ameliorative measures applied. The suggestion of an overlap between the child vulnerable to a hospital stay and those from disadvantaged homes makes this even more important.

(ii) Research is needed into the circumstances and consequences of repeat admissions, to isolate the special strains involved and again because of possible connections with chronic disadvantage.

(iii) Work about discontinuity and its meaning for children should be extended in a variety of ways. Detailed psychological work should be extended to the 6-11 group which fell between the work of Brown and Clough: further sociological work is needed in the teenage group. There is need to validate Clough's complex and important findings on another population, on different treatment categories and on boys as well as girls.

(iv) A longitudinal study of handicapped children and their parents could provide much-needed insight and under-standing. All studies to date have been cross-sectional.

(v) The developments which follow health circular HC(76)5 which recommends that nurses be trained to play with children as part of their nursing duties should be carefully surveyed.

(vi) There is a variety of styles of play with different aims. Before any one method is established routinely throughout the nursing profession, there is need for research to establish the implications of each of these. Perhaps such research should go alongside the initial attempts to implement HC(76)5.

(vii) We have recommended that the emotional needs of staff should be recognised and handled. Research is needed to establish how this could best be done. This implies an examination of the traditional methods of control and the exploration of alternative methods in light of the need to maintain high discipline in the treatment situation.

(viii) Paediatricians and other consultants may wish to experiment with ameliorative measures in their wards. There is a case for co-operative work to assess these.

(ix) The progress of any seminars which are set up to

work through some of the findings of this research with
practitioners in practical situations could also be
carefully watched, for they could become the model for
the application of other psychological or sociological
findings to therapy.

(x) There may be a case for developing child-patient
registers similar to the psychiatric registers. These
would make it possible to monitor the use of child-health
services in a given area and to explore some of the
propositions about treatment careers and the influence of
social variables. Such a register would provide a basis
for the identification of sub-samples (e.g. repeat
admissions) for further research. They could be an
effective tool in the evaluation of the child health
service.

(xi) It is clear that much of what has been said in
this volume has implications for the treatment of many
categories of patients other than children, and indicates
the need for research specific to such other areas.
Details of that research will not be indicated here.
Those who are interested will undoubtedly be able to
draw their own parallels.

Notes

CHAPTER 5 DEMANDS AND RESPONSES

1 At intervals throughout the day, information about the position, activities and interactions of each child was entered on a pre-coded sheet. It included any visitors or staff who were present as potential or actual partners in interaction. Details of the activity-sampling and other research methods may be found in Hall (1977).

2 Basic and technical procedures were recorded roughly in the proportions 7:3 during the three weeks; that is, basic procedures, which concern food, cleanliness and comfort, were observed more than twice as often as the more technical. This lends force to the picture suggested by the distribution of sightings.

3 Case studies refer to children who were observed continuously for five minutes in each hour, 16 hours a day, throughout their stay in the ward.

4 This account is taken from Hall and Cleary (1974). The bed positions of the participants are marked on the plan of the ward (see Figure 5.1).

5 These first two extracts include reference to Judith on the day of admission and on the fourth day of her stay. The remaining extracts are selected as illustrative of the way in which she handled during her period of stay in the ward.

CHAPTER 6 STATUS AND CAREER

1 Illness behaviour is the process by which pain and symptoms are defined, accorded significance and socially labelled, help is sought, changes in the life regimen brought about and claims are made on others (Mechanic, 1968).

2   Twaddle (1974) argues that the process of health-status
    designation 'consists of interaction between an indi-
    vidual and his status definers in which normative
    standards of adequacy are applied to the individual in
    the context of a specific situation to assess his
    capacities for present or future role and task
    performance'.
3   Health status may, of course, change radically over
    time as the result of illness or trauma.
4   The DHSS itself commissioned a survey (DHSS, 1970), and
    the issues have been discussed in several of the annual
    reports, notably for 1966, 1967 and 1970.
5   The base used is taken from *Report on the Census of
    Children and Adolescents in Non-Psychiatric Wards in
    N.H.S. Hospitals,* June 1964 and March 1965, Ministry
    of Health, Statistical Report Series No. 2, HMSO, 1967.
    The total number of children aged 0-15 on 24 March 1965
    was 19,468.
6   Cf. Hospital Inpatient Enquiry 1967, Table 13.
7   This theme is developed more fully in Pill (1976).
8   Post-hospital behavioural disturbance was measured using
    three methods (a) by direct questioning of the mother
    on changes in the child's behaviour, (b) a questionnaire
    developed by Vernon et al. (1966) completed by the
    mothers (this measured six dimensions: general anxiety
    and repression; separation anxiety; sleep anxiety;
    eating disturbance; aggression towards authority;
    apathy - withdrawal), (c) the Bristol Social Adjustment
    Guide, completed by the child's teacher (Stott, 1971).

Bibliography

ABEL-SMITH, B. (1964), 'The Hospitals: 1800-1948'. London: Heinemann.

AINSWORTH, M.D.S (1969), Object Relations, Dependency and Attachment: A Theoretical Review of Infant-Mother Relationship, 'Child Development', 40, 969-1025.

ANDERSON, O.W. and ANDERSEN, R.M. (1972), Patterns of Use of Health Services, in H.E Freeman, S. Levine and L.G. Reader (eds), 'Handbook of Medical Sociology'. (2nd edn), Englewood Cliffs: Prentice Hall.

BAKKE, K. (1974), Primary Nursing, 'American Journal of Nursing', 74, 1432-4.

BARKER, R.G., WRIGHT, B.A., MYERSON, L. and GONICK, M.R (1953), 'Adjustment to Physical Handicap and Illness', Bulletin 55 (revd edn), New York: Social Science Research Council.

BECKER, H.S. (1963), 'Outsiders', New York: Free Press.

BENE, E. and ANTHONY, J. (1957), 'Manual for the Family Relations Test', London: National Foundation for Educational Research.

BENNETT, A.E., GARRAD, J. and HALIL, T. (1970), Chronic Disease and Disability in the Community: A Prevalence Study, 'British Medical Journal', 3, 762-4.

BERLYNE, D.E. (1965), 'Structure and Direction in Thinking', New York: Wiley.

BION, W.R. (1961), 'Experiences in Groups', London: Tavistock.

BLAU, P.M. (1964), 'Exchange and Power in Social Life', New York: Wiley.

BLOOR, M.J. and HOROBIN, G.W. (1975), Conflict and Conflict Resolution in Doctor/Patient Interactions, in C. Cox and A. Mead (eds), 'A Sociology of Medical Practice', London: Collier Macmillan.

BLUMER, H. (1969), 'Symbolic Interactionism', Englewood Cliffs: Prentice-Hall.

BOSSARD, J.H.S. and BOLL, E.S. (1960), 'The Sociology of
Child Development', New York: Harper.
BOWLBY, J. (1952), 'Maternal Care and Mental Health' (2nd
edn), Geneva: World Health Organization.
BOWLBY, J. (1960), Separation Anxiety, 'International
Journal of Psycho-Analysis', 41, 69-113
BOWLBY, J. (1961), Processes of Mourning, 'International
Journal of Psycho-Analysis', 42, 318-40.
BOWLBY, J. (1968), Effects on Behaviour of Disruption of
an Affectional Bond, in J.M. Thoday and A.S. Parkes (eds),
'Genetic and Environmental Influences on Behaviour',
Edinburgh: Oliver & Boyd.
BOWLBY, J. (1969), 'Attachment', London: Hogarth.
BRAIN, D.J. and MACLAY, I. (1968), Controlled Study of
Mothers and Children in Hospital, 'British Medical Journal',
1, 278-80.
BRITTAN, A. (1973), 'Meanings and Situations', London:
Routledge & Kegan Paul.
BRONFENBRENNER, U. (1970), 'Two Worlds of Childhood:
US and USSR', New York: Russell Sage Foundation.
BROWN, B.J. (1977), Some Aspects of the Responses of Young
Children to Separation and Strange Situations: A Study
of Individual Differences, unpublished PhD thesis,
University of Wales.
BROWN, G.W. (1973), The Mental Hospital as an Institution,
'Social Science and Medicine', 7, 407-24.
BUCHER, R. and STRAUSS, A. (1960), Professions in Process,
'American Journal of Sociology', 66, 325-34.
BURNS, T. and STALKER, G.M (1961), 'The Management of
Innovation', London: Tavistock.
BURTON, L. (1975), 'The Family Life of Sick Children',
London: Routledge & Kegan Paul.
CAMPBELL, E.H. (1957), Effects of Mothers' Anxiety on
Infants' Behaviour, unpublished PhD thesis, Yale University.
CAMPBELL, J.D. (1975), Illness is a Point of View: The
Development of Children's Concepts of Illness, 'Child
Development', 46, 92-100.
CARTWRIGHT, A. (1964), 'Human Relations and Hospital Care',
London: Routledge & Kegan Paul.
CASSEE, E. (1975), Therapeutic Behaviour, Hospital Culture
and Communication, in C. Cox and A. Mead (eds), 'A
Sociology of Medical Practice', London: Collier Macmillan.
CAUDILL, W.F. (1958), 'The Psychiatric Hospital as a
Small Society', Cambridge: Harvard University Press.
CENTERS, L. and CENTERS, R. (1963), Peer Group Attitudes
Toward the Amputee Child, 'Journal of Social Psychology',
61, 127-32.
CICOUREL, A.V. (1964), 'Method and Measurement in
Sociology', New York: Free Press.

CLARKE, A.M. and CLARKE, A.D.B. (1976), 'Early Experience: Myth and Evidence', London: Open Books.

CLOUGH, F. (1973), 'Cognitive Developmental Theory and the Hospitalisation of Children', paper read to British Psychological Society Conference, Liverpool (mimeo).

CLOUGH, F. (1975), 'Two Studies of Older Children in Hospital', report to the Department of Health and Social Security (mimeo), Medical Sociology Research Centre, University of Swansea.

COE, R.M. (1970), 'Sociology of Medicine', New York: McGraw-Hill.

COLEMAN, L.L. (1950), The Psychological Implications of Tonsillectomy, 'New York Journal of Medicine', 50, 1225-8.

COOLEY, W.W. and LOHNES, P.R. (1971), 'Multivariate Data Analysis', New York: Wiley.

COOMBS, R.H. and GOLDMAN, L.J. (1973), Maintenance and Discontinuity of Coping Mechanisms in an Intensive Care Unit, 'Social Problems', 20, 342-55.

COSER, R.L. (1963), Alienation and the Social Structure: Case Analysis of a Hospital, in E. Freidson (ed.), 'The Hospital in Modern Society', London: Collier Macmillan.

COSER, R.L. (1976a), Suicide and Reactional System: A Case Study in a Mental Hospital, 'Journal of Health and Social Behavior', 17, 318-27,

COSER, R.L. (1976b), Stay Home, Little Sheba: On Placement, Displacement and Social Change, 'Social Problems', 22, 470-80.

COURT, D. and JACKSON, A. (1972), 'Paediatrics in the Seventies', Occasional Hundreds 4, London: Oxford University Press.

CROSS, K.W. and TURNER, R.D. (1974), Patient Visiting and the Siting of Hospitals in Rural Areas, 'British Journal of Preventive and Social Medicine', 28, 276-80.

DAVIE, R., BUTLER, N. and GOLDSTEIN, H. (1972), 'From Birth to Seven', second report of the National Child Development Study, London: Longmans.

DAVIES, C. (1972), Professionals in Organisations: Some Preliminary Observations on Hospital Consultants, 'Sociological Review', 20, 553-67.

DAVIES, C. (1976), Experiences of Dependency and Control in Work: The Case of Nurses, 'Journal of Advanced Nursing', 1, 1-10.

DAVIES, C. and FRANCIS, A. (1976), Perceptions of Structure in NHS Hospitals, in M. Stacey (ed.), 'The Sociology of the National Health Service', Sociological Review Monograph 22, University of Keele.

DAVIS, F. (1960), Uncertainty in Medical Prognosis, Clinical and Functional, 'American Journal of Sociology', 66, 41-7.

DAVIS, F. (1963), 'Passage Through Crisis', Indianapolis:
Bobbs-Merrill.
DAVIS, F. (1975), Professional Socialisation as Subjective
Experience: The Process of Doctrinal Conversion Among
Student Nurses, in C. Cox and A. Mead (eds), 'A Sociology
of Medical Practice', London: Collier Macmillan.
DEARDEN, R. (1970), The Psychiatric Aspects of the Case-
Study Sample, in M. Stacey, R. Dearden, R. Pill and
D. Robinson, 'Hospitals, Children and their Families',
London: Routledge & Kegan Paul.
DELIEGE, D. and LEROY, X. (1975), 'L'assistance psycho-
sociale à l'hôpital', conference paper, Ecole de Santé
publique (U.C.L).
DE MARSH, K.G and MCLELLAN, E.I. (1971), Nurses Sold on a
Shortened Working Week, 'Canadian Hospital', 48, 64-6.
DENZIN, N.K. (1970), 'The Research Act in Sociology',
London: Butterworths.
DEPARTMENT OF HEALTH AND SOCIAL SECURITY (1969) 'Report
of the Committee of Enquiry into Allegations of Ill-
Treatment of Patients and Other Irregularities at the Ely
Hospital, Cardiff', (Cmnd 3975), London: HMSO.
DEPARTMENT OF HEALTH AND SOCIAL SECURITY (1970), 'The
Report on the Survey of Long-Stay Hospital Accommodation
for Children', London: DHSS (mimeo).
DEPARTMENT OF HEALTH AND SOCIAL SECURITY (1972), 'Report
of the Committee on Nursing' (Briggs Report) (Cmnd 5115),
London: HMSO.
DEPARTMENT OF HEALTH AND SOCIAL SECURITY (1976a), 'Report
of the Expert Group on Play for Children in Hospital',
published with 'Play for Children in Hospital' (Circular
HC (76)5), London: HMSO.
DEPARTMENT OF HEALTH AND SOCIAL SECURITY (1976b), 'Fit
for the Future', report of the Committee on Child Health
Services (Court Report), London: HMSO.
DEPARTMENT OF HEALTH AND SOCIAL SECURITY and OFFICE OF
POPULATION CENSUSES AND SURVEYS (1974), 'Report on
Hospital In-Patient Enquiry, 1972,' London: HMSO.
DODD, A.P. (1973), Towards an Understanding of Nursing,
unpublished PhD thesis, University of London.
DOUGLAS, J.W.B. (1975), Early Hospital Admissions and
Later Disturbances of Behaviour and Learning, 'Develop-
mental Medicine and Child Neurology', 17, 456-80.
DOUGLAS, J.W.B. LAWSON, A., COOPER, J.E. and COOPER, E.
(1968), Family Interaction and the Activities of Young
Children, 'Journal of Child Psychology and Psychiatry',
9, 157-71.
DOUGLAS, M. (1966), 'Purity and Danger', London: Routledge
& Kegan Paul.
DUBOS, R. (1968), 'Man, Medicine and Environment',
Harmondsworth: Penguin.

DUFF, R.S. and HOLLINGSHEAD, A.B. (1968), 'Sickness and Society', New York: Harper & Row.

EDELSTON, H. (1943), Separation Anxiety in Young Children, 'Genetic Psychology Monographs', 28, 3-95.

ETHERINGTON, A. (1970), Team Nursing in the U.S.A., 'Nursing Times', 66, 110-12.

ETZIONI, A. (1961), 'A Comparative Analysis of Complex Organisations', New York: Free Press.

ETZIONI, A. (ed.) (1969), 'The Semi-Professions and their Organisation', New York: Free Press.

EVANS-PRITCHARD, E.E. (1937), 'Witchcraft, Oracles and Magic among the Azande', Oxford: Clarendon Press.

EVANS-PRITCHARD, E.E. (1956), 'Nuer Religion', Oxford: Clarendon Press.

EYSENCK, H.J. (1952), 'The Scientific Study of Personality', London: Routledge & Kegan Paul.

FEATHER, N.T. (1963), Mowrer's Revised Two-Factor Theory and the Motive-Expectancy-Value Model, 'Psychological Review', 70, 500-15.

FESTINGER, L. (1954), A Theory of Social Comparison Processes, 'Human Relations', 7, 117-40.

FESTINGER, L. (1957), 'A Theory of Cognitive Dissonance', Evanston: Row, Peterson.

FOOTE, N.N. and COTTRELL Jnr, L.S. (1955), 'Identity and Interpersonal Competence', Chicago: University of Chicago Press.

FOUCAULT, M. (1967), 'Madness and Civilisation', London: Tavistock.

FOUCAULT, M. (1973), 'The Birth of the Clinic', London: Tavistock.

FOX, R.C. (1975), Training for Uncertainty, in C. Cox and A. Mead (eds), 'A Sociology of Medical Practice', London: Collier Macmillan.

FREIDSON, E. (1961), 'Patients' Views of Medical Practice', New York: Russell Sage Foundation.

FREIDSON, E. (1965), Disability as Social Deviance, in M. Susser (ed.), 'Sociology and Rehabilitation', Washington DC: American Sociological Association.

FREIDSON, E. (1970), 'Profession of Medicine', New York: Dodds, Mead.

FREIDSON, E. (1975), Dilemmas in the Doctor/Patient Relationship, in C. Cox and A. Mead (eds), 'A Sociology of Medical Practice', London: Collier Macmillan.

GEERTZ, C. (1964), Ideology as a Cultural System, in D.E. Apter (ed.), 'Ideology and Discontent', New York: Free Press.

GLASER, W.A. (1970), 'Social Settings and Medical Organisation', New York: Atherton.

GLUCKMAN, M. (1965), 'Politics, Law and Ritual in Tribal Society', Oxford: Blackwell.

GOFFMAN, E. (1961), 'Asylums', New York: Doubleday.
GOFFMAN, E. (1963), 'Stigma', Englewood Cliffs: Prentice-Hall.
GOFFMAN, E. (1971), 'The Presentation of Self in Everyday Life', Harmondsworth: Penguin (first published 1959).
GOLDSTEIN, J., FREUD, A. and SOLNIT, A.J. (1973), 'Beyond the Best Interests of the Child', New York: Free Press.
GOSLIN, D.A. (ed.) (1969), 'Handbook of Socialisation Theory and Research', Chicago: Rand McNally.
GORDON, B. (1973), Children in Hospital: An Inter-disciplinary Approach to the Sick Child and His Family, paper presented to the British Psychology Society conference, Liverpool.
GORDON, B. (1974), An Interdisciplinary Approach to the Dying Child and His Family, in L. Burton (ed.), 'Care of the Child Facing Death', London: Routledge & Kegan Paul.
HALES-TOOKE, A. (1973), 'Children in Hospital: The Parents' View', London: Priory Press.
HALL, D. and CLEARY, J. (1974), 'The Hospital Playleader Project', Report to the Department of Health and Social Security, Medical Sociology Research Centre, University College of Swansea (mimeo).
HALL, D.J.,PILL, R. and CLOUGH, F. (1976), Notes for a Conceptual Model of Hospital Experience as an Interactive Process, in M. Stacey (ed.), 'The Sociology of the National Health Service', Sociological Review Monograph 22, University of Keele.
HALL, D.J. (1977), 'Social Relations and Innovation', London: Routledge & Kegan Paul.
HALL, O. (1948), The Stages of a Medical Career, 'American Journal of Sociology', 53, 327-36.
HARRISSON, S. (1974), A Matter of Routine, 'Nursing Times', 70, September, Occasional Paper.
HARRISSON, S.P. (1975), Social Consequences of the Long Term Medical Treatment of Children, unpublished DPhil thesis, University of York.
HARVEY, O.J. (ed.) (1963), 'Motivation and Social Interaction', New York: Ronald Press.
HAWTHORN, P.J. (1974), 'Nurse - I Want My Mummy!', London: Royal College of Nursing.
HERBERT, G.W. (1974), Teachers' Ratings of Classroom Behaviour: Factorial Structure, 'British Journal of Educational Psychology', 44, 233-40.
HERZLICH, C. (1973), 'Health and Illness', European Monographs in Social Psychology 5, London: Academic Press.
HEWITT, S. (1970), 'The Family and the Handicapped Child', London: Allen & Unwin.
HEWETT, S. (1972),'The Need for Long-Term Care',

Occasional Paper 3, Institute for Research into Mental
Retardation, London: Butterworths.
HUGHES, E.C. (1958), 'Men and Their Work', Chicago:
Free Press.
ILLICH, I. (1975), 'Medical Nemesis', London: Calder &
Boyars.
INHELDER, B. and PIAGET, J. (1958), 'The Growth of
Logical Thinking from Childhood to Adolescence', London:
Routledge & Kegan Paul.
INKELES, A. (1966), Social Structure and the Socialisation
of Competence, 'Harvard Educational Review', 36, 3.
JAMES, V.L. and WHEELER, W.E. (1969), The Care-by-Parent
Unit, 'Pediatrics', 43, 488-94.
JAQUES, E. (1956), Social Systems as a Defence Against
Persecutory and Depressive Anxiety, in M. Klein, P. Heimann
and R.E. Money-Kyrle (eds), 'New Directions in Psycho-
analysis', London: Tavistock.
JESSNER, L., BLOM, G.E. and WALDFOGEL, S. (1952),
Emotional Implications of Tonsillectomy and Adenoidectomy
on Children, 'Psychoanalytic Study of the Child', 7,
New York: International Universities Press.
JOHNSON, M.M. and MARTIN, H.W. (1965), A Sociological
Analysis of the Nurse Role, in J.K. Skipper and R.C.
Leonard (eds), 'Social Interaction and Patient Care',
Philadelphia: Lippincott.
JOLLY, J.D. (1974), The Ward Granny System, 'Nursing
Times', 70, 537-40.
JONES, K. (1975), 'Opening the Door', London: Routledge
& Kegan Paul.
KALVERBOER, A.F. (1971), Observation of Exploratory
Behaviour of Pre-School Children Alone and in the Presence
of the Mother, 'Psychiatria Neurologia Neurochirurgia',
74, 43-57.
KATZ, S., JACKSON, B.A., JAFFE, M.W., LITTELL, A.S. and
TURK, C.E. (1958), Multidisciplinary Studies of Illness
in Aged Persons. (1) Methods and Results, 'Journal of
Chronic Diseases', 7, 332-6.
KELVIN, P. (1969), 'The Bases of Social Behaviour',
New York: Holt Rinehart & Winston.
KING, R.D., RAYNES, N.V. and TIZARD, J. (1971), 'Patterns
of Residential Care', London: Routledge & Kegan Paul.
KNUTSON, A.L. (1965), 'The Individual, Society and Health
Behaviour', New York: Russell Sage Foundation.
KOOS, E.L. (1954), 'The Health of Regionville', New York:
Columbia University Press.
LADYBIRD (1963), 'People at Work. The Nurse', Lough-
borough: Ladybird.
LAWRIE, R. (1964), Operating on Children as Day Cases,
'Lancet', 2, 1289-91.

LERNER, M.J., HALEY, J.V., HALL, D.S. and McVARISH, D.
(1972), Hospital Care-by-Parent: An Evaluative Look,
'Medical Care', 10, 430-6.
LEWIS, A. (1953), Health as a Social Concept, 'British
Journal of Sociology', 4, 109-24.
LORBER, J. (1975), Good Patients and Problem Patients:
Conformity and Deviance in a General Hospital, 'Journal
of Health and Social Behaviour', 16, 213-25.
MacCARTHY, D. (1957), Mothers in Hospital with Their
Children, 'Public Health', 71, 264.
MacCARTHY, D., LINDSAY, H. and MORRIS, I. (1962),
Children in Hospital with Their Mothers, 'Lancet', 1,
603-8.
MacCARTHY, D. (1974), Communication Between Children and
Doctors, 'Developmental Medicine and Child Neurology', 16,
279-85.
MacGUIRE, J.M. (1968), The Function of the 'Set' in
Hospital Controlled Schemes of Nurse Training, 'British
Journal of Sociology', 19, 271-83.
MACINTYRE, S. (1977), Old Age as a Social Problem:
Historical Notes on the English Experience, in R. Dingwall,
C. Heath, M. Reid and M. Stacey (eds), 'Health Care and
Health Knowledge', London: Croom Helm.
MAIN, T.F. (1968), The Ailment, in E. Barnes (ed.)
'Psychosocial Nursing', London: Tavistock.
MAPES, R.E.A. and ALLEN, G.J.B. (1973), Path Analysis -
A Cautionary Note, 'Sociological Review', 21, 137-44.
MARRAM, G.D., SCHLEGEL, M.W. and BEVIS, E.O. (1974),
'Primary Nursing', St Louis: Mosby.
MAUKSCH, H.O. (1973), Ideology, Interaction and Patient
Care in Hospitals, 'Social Science and Medicine', 7, 817-30.
McELNEA, L. (1971), Where Resident Parents are Welcome,
'Nursing Times', 67, 1331-3.
McHUGH, P. (1968), 'Defining the Situation', Indianapolis:
Bobbs-Merrill.
McMICHAEL, J.K. (1971), 'Handicap', London: Staples Press.
MECHANIC, D. (1968), 'Medical Sociology', New York: Free
Press.
MENZIES, I.E.P. (1960), A Case-Study in the Functioning
of Social Systems as a Defence Against Anxiety, 'Human
Relations', 13,95-121.
MERTON, R.K. (1957), 'Social Theory and Social Structure'
(revd edn), New York: Free Press.
MERTON, R.K., READER, G.G. and KENDALL, P.L. (eds) (1957),
'The Student-Physician', Cambridge: Harvard University
Press.
MILLER, E.J. and GWYNNE, G.V. (1972), 'A Life Apart',
London: Tavistock.
MILLER, E.J. and GWYNNE, G.V (1973), Dependence, Indepen-

dence and Counter-Dependence in Residential Institutions for Incurables, in R. Gosling (ed.), 'Support, Innovation and Autonomy', Tavistock Clinic Golden Jubilee Paper, London: Tavistock.

MILLER, E.J. and RICE, A.K. (1967), 'Systems of Organisation', London: Tavistock.

MINISTRY OF HEALTH (1959), 'The Welfare of Children in Hospital' (Platt Report), London: HMSO.

MINISTRY OF HEALTH (1966), 'Report of the Committee on Senior Nursing Staff Structure' (Salmon Report), London: HMSO.

MINISTRY OF HEALTH (1967), 'On the State of Public Health 1966', Annual Report of the Chief Medical Officer of the Ministry of Health, London: HMSO.

MOORE, T. (1969), Stress in Normal Childhood, 'Human Relations', 22, 235-50.

NATIONAL ASSOCIATION FOR THE WELFARE OF CHILDREN IN HOSPITAL (1975), 'Survey of Visiting and Parents' Accommodation', London: NAWCH (mimeo).

NEW, P.K.-M., NITE, G. and CALLAHAN, J. (1965), Too Many Nurses May Be Worse Than Too Few, in J.K. Skipper and R.C. Leonard (eds), 'Social Interaction and Patient Care', Philadelphia: Lippincott.

NEWSON, J. and NEWSON, E. (1965), 'Patterns of Infant Care in an Urban Community', Harmondsworth: Penguin (first published 1963).

NIGHTINGALE, F. (1859), 'Notes on Nursing', London: Harrison.

NOBLE, E. (1967), 'Play and the Sick Child', London: Faber.

OPPE, T.E. (1971), Home Care for Sick Children,'British Journal of Hospital Medicine', 5, 39-44.

ORNSTEIN, R.E. (1969), 'On the Experience of Time', Harmondsworth: Penguin.

OSGOOD, C.E.,SUCI, G.J. and TANNENBAUM, P.H. (1957), 'The Measurement of Meaning', Illinois: University of Illinois Press.

OSWIN, M. (1971), 'The Empty Hours', London: Allen Lane.

PACKMAN, J. and POWER, M. (1968), Children in Need and the Help They Receive, Appendix Q, 'Report of the Committee on Local Authority and Allied Personal Social Services' (Seebohm Report) (Cmnd 3703), London: HMSO.

PARSONS, T. (1951), 'The Social System', London: Routledge & Kegan Paul.

PARSONS, T. (1958), Definitions of Health and Illness in the Light of American Values and Social Structure, in E.G. Jaco (ed.), 'Patients, Physicians and Illness', New York: Free Press.

PERROW, C. (1963), Goals and Power Structures - A

Historical Case Study, in E. Freidson (ed.), 'The Hospital in Modern Society', New York: Free Press.

PERROW, C. (1965), Hospitals: Technology, Structure and Goals, in J.G. March (ed.), 'Handbook of Organisations', Chicago: Rand McNally.

PETRILLO, M. and SANGER, S. (1972), 'Emotional Care of Hospitalised Children', Philadelphia: Lippincott.

PIAGET, J. (1967), 'Six Psychological Studies', New York: Random House (first published 1964).

PILL, R.M. (1967), A Social Study of the Hospitalisation of Young Children, unpublished MSc (Econ.) thesis, University of Wales.

PILL, R.M. (1976), Health Careers and Competence: Aspects of Behaviour on a Children's Ward, 'Social Science and Medicine', 10, 105-11.

PILL, R. with JACOBS, R. (1974), 'Report on a Pilot Study on the Problems of Long-Stay Children in Hospital', Report to the Department of Health and Social Security, Medical Sociology Research Centre, University College of Swansea (mimeo).

PLANK, E.N. (1964), 'Working with Children in Hospitals', London: Tavistock.

PRINGLE, M.L.K. (1964), 'The Emotional and Social Adjustment of Physically Handicapped Children', Occasional Publication 11, Slough: National Foundation for Educational Research.

PRUGH, D.G., STAUB, E.M., SANDS, H.H., KIRSCHBAUM, R.M. and LENIHAN, E.A. (1953), A Study of the Emotional Reactions of Children and Families to Hospitalisation and Illness, 'American Journal of Orthopsychiatry', 23, 70-106.

QUAY, H.C. and QUAY, L.C. (1965), Behaviour Problems in Early Adolescence, 'Child Development', 36, 215-20.

REVANS, R.W. (1964), 'Standards for Morale', London: Oxford University Press.

RICHARDSON, S.A., GOODMAN, N., HASTORF, A.H. and DORNBUSCH, S.M. (1961), Cultural Uniformity in Reaction to Physical Disabilities, 'American Sociological Review', 26, 241-7.

RICHARDSON, S.A. (1969), The Effect of Physical Disability on the Socialisation of a Child, in D.A. Gosling (ed.), 'Handbook of Socialisation Theory and Research', Chicago: Rand MacNally.

RILEY, I.D., SYME, J., HALL, M.S. and PATRICK, M.J. (1975), Mother and Child in Hospital - Two Years' Experience, 'British Medical Journal', 2, 990-2.

ROBB, B. (1967), 'Sans Everything', London: Nelson.

ROBERTSON, J. (1953), Some Responses of Young Children to Loss of Maternal Care, 'Nursing Times', 49, 382-6.

ROBERTSON, J. (1959), A Two-Year-Old Goes to Hospital,

'Guide to the Film', London: Tavistock.

ROBERTSON, J. (1960), The Plight of Small Children in Hospital, 'Parents' Magazine', June.

ROBERTSON, J. (1970), 'Young Children in Hospital' (2nd edn), London: Tavistock.

ROBINSON, D.A. (1967), Some Aspects of the Attitudes and Behaviour of Parents in Relation to the Hospitalisation of their Young Children, unpublished PhD thesis, University of Wales.

ROBINSON, D. (1970), The Social Milieu, in M. Stacey, R. Dearden, R. Pill and D. Robinson, 'Hospitals, Children and Their Families', London: Routledge & Kegan Paul.

ROBINSON, D. (1971), 'The Process of Becoming Ill', London: Routledge & Kegan Paul.

ROBOTTOM, B.M. (1969), The Contribution of the Children's Nurse to the Home Care of Children, 'British Journal of Medical Education', 3, 311-12.

ROSENBERG, M. and PEARLIN, L.I. (1962), Power-Orientations in the Mental Hospital, 'Human Relations', 15, 335-49.

ROSENGREN, W.R. and LEFTON, M. (1969), 'Hospitals and Patients', New York: Atherton.

ROTH, J.A. (1963), 'Timetables', Indianapolis, Bobbs-Merrill.

RUTTER, M. (1972), 'Maternal Deprivation Reassessed', Harmondsworth: Penguin.

RUTTER, M. and MITTLER, P. (1972), Environmental Influences on Language Development, in M. Rutter and J.A.M. Martin (eds), 'The Child with Delayed Speech', London: Heinemann.

SCHAFFER, H.R. and CALLENDER, W.M. (1959), Psychologic Effects of Hospitalisation in Infancy, 'Pediatrics', 24, 528-39.

SCHUMACHER, E.F. (1973), 'Small Is Beautiful', London: Blond & Briggs.

SELLORS, T.H. and RAINS, A.J.H. (1975), What Is a Hospital For?, 'World Medicine', 10, 54-63.

SHAPIRO, M.B. (1961), A Method of Measuring Psychological Changes Specific to the Individual Psychiatric Patient, 'British Journal of Medical Psychology', 34, 151-5.

SILVERMAN, D. (1970), 'The Theory of Organisation', London: Heinemann.

SKIPPER, J.K. and LEONARD, R.C. (eds) (1965), 'Social Interaction and Patient Care', Philadelphia: Lippincott.

SPENCE, J.C. (1946), 'The Purpose of the Family', London: Tavistock.

SPENCE, J.C. (1947), The Care of Children in Hospital, 'British Medical Journal', 1, 125-30.

SPENCE, J.C. (1951), Children in Hospital with Their Mothers, 'American Journal of Nursing', 51, 14.

STACEY, M., DEARDEN, R., PILL, R. and ROBINSON, D. (1970),

'Hospitals, Children and Their Families', London: Routledge & Kegan Paul.

STACEY, M. and EARTHROWL, B. (1973), 'Children in Hospital in Wales: The Report of a Survey for the Welsh Hospital Board', Medical Sociology Research Centre, University College of Swansea (mimeo).

STACEY, M. (1976), The Health Service Consumer: A Sociological Misconception, in M. Stacey (ed.) 'The Sociology of the National Health Service', Sociological Monograph 22, University of Keele.

STANTON, A.H. and SCHWARTZ, M.S. (1954), 'The Mental Hospital', New York: Basic Books.

STAPLES, S. and CURTIS, B.L. (1975), Extended Work Day - Two Tears Later, 'Hospital Administration in Canada', 17, 32-4.

STEBBINS, R.A. (1971), The Meaning of Disorderly Behaviour; Teacher Definitions of a Classroom Situation, 'Sociology of Education', 44, 217-36.

STEVENS, R. (1966), 'Medical Practice in Modern England', New Haven: Yale University Press.

STEWART, R. and SLEEMAN, J. (1967), 'Continuously Under Review', Occasional Paper on Social Administration 20, London: Bell.

STIMSON, G.V. (1974), Obeying Doctors' Orders: A View From the Other Side, 'Social Science and Medicine', 8, 97-104.

STIMSON, G. and WEBB, B. (1975), 'Going to See the Doctor', London: Routledge & Kegan Paul.

STIMSON, G.V. (1976), General Practitioners, 'Trouble' and Types of Patients, in M. Stacey (ed.), 'The Sociology of the National Health Service', Sociological Review Monograph 22, University of Keele.

STOCKWELL, F. (1972), 'The Unpopular Patient', London: Royal College of Nursing.

STOTT, D.H. (1971), 'The Social Adjustment of Children' (manual to the Bristol Social Adjustment Guides), London: University of London Press (first published 1958).

STRAUSS, A.L. (1956), 'The Social Psychology of George Herbert Mead', Chicago: University of Chicago Press.

STRAUSS, A., SCHATZMAN, L., EHRLICH, D., BUCHER, R. and SABSHIN, M. (1963), The Hospital and Its Negotiated Order, in E. Freidson (ed.), 'The Hospital in Modern Society', London: Collier Macmillan.

SUCHMAN, E.A. (1964), Sociomedical Variations Among Ethnic Groups, 'American Journal of Sociology', 70, 319-31.

SUCHMAN, E.A. (1965a), Social Patterns of Illness and Medical Care, 'Journal of Health and Human Behaviour', 6, 2-16.

SUCHMAN, E.A. (1965b), Stages of Illness and Medical Care,

'Journal of Health and Human Behaviour', 6, 114-28.
TAYLOR, C. (1970), 'In Horizontal Orbit', New York:
Holt, Rinehart & Winston.
TIZARD, J., SINCLAIR, I. and CLARKE, R.V.G. (eds) (1975),
'Varieties of Residential Experience', London: Routledge
& Kegan Paul.
TOPLISS, E.P. (1974), Organisational Change as Illustrated
by a Case-Study of a Geriatric Hospital, 'British Journal
of Sociology', 25, 356-66.
TOWELL, D. (1975), 'Understanding Psychiatric Nursing',
London: Royal College of Nursing.
TURNER, R.H. (1962), Role-Taking: Process Versus Con-
formity, in A.M. Rose (ed.), 'Human Behaviour and Social
Processes', London: Routledge & Kegan Paul.
TWADDLE, A.C. (1974), The Concept of Health Status,
'Social Science and Medicine', 8, 29-38.
VAN GENNEP (1960), 'The Rites of Passage', London:
Routledge & Kegan Paul (first published 1908).
VEENEKLAAS, G.M.H. (1976), Psychosocial Teaching in the
Leiden Paediatric Department, unpublished paper,
University of Leiden.
VERNON, D.T.A., BOLEY, J.M., SIPOWICZ, R.R. and SCHULMAN,
J.L. (1965), 'The Psychological Responses of Children to
Hospitalisation and Illness', Springfield: Thomas.
VERNON, D.T.A., FOLEY, J.M. and SCHULMAN, J.L. (1966),
Changes in Children's Behaviour Following Hospitalisation:
Some Dimensions of Response and Their Correlates,
'American Journal of Diseases of Children', 3, 581-93.
VOYSEY, M. (1975), 'A Constant Burden', London: Routledge
& Kegan Paul.
WAITZKIN, H. and STOECKLE, J.D. (1972), The Communication
of Information About Illness: Clinical, Sociological and
Methodological Considerations, 'Advances in Psychosomatic
Medicine', 8, 180-215.
WAITZKIN, H. with STOECKLE, J.D. (1976), Information
Control and the Micropolitics of Health Care: Summary
of an Ongoing Research Project, 'Social Science and Medicine',
10, 263-76.
WEBB, B. (1977), Trauma and Tedium: An Account of Living-
In on a Children's Ward, in A. Davis and G. Horobin,
'Medical Encounters', London: Croom Helm.
WEINICK, J.R. (1958), Psychological Study of Emotional
Reaction of Children to Tonsillectomy, unpublished PhD
thesis, University of New York.
WEINSTEIN, E.A. (1969), The Development of Interpersonal
Competence, in D.A. Goslin (ed.), 'Handbook of
Socialisation Theory and Research', Chicago: Rand McNally.
WELSH HOSPITAL BOARD (1972), 'Children in Hospital in
Wales', final report of the working party, Cardiff: WHB.

WEST, P. (1977), The Epileptic Career: The Role of the
Runaway Doctor, in M. Wadsworth and D. Robinson (eds),
'Studies in Everyday Medical Life', London: Martin
Robertson.
WHEELER, S. (1966), The Structure of Formally Organised
Socialisation Settings, in O.G. Brim and S. Wheeler,
'Socialisation After Childhood', New York: Wiley.
WINNICOTT, D.W. (1971), 'Therapeutic Consultations in
Child Psychiatry', London: Hogarth Press.
WOODWARD, J. (1959), Emotional Disturbances of Burned
Children, 'British Medical Journal', 1, 1009-13.
WOODWARD, J. (1962), Parental Visiting of Children with
Burns, 'British Medical Journal', 2, 1656-7.
YARROW, L.J. (1964), Separation from Parents During Early
Childhood, in M.L. Hoffman and L.W. Hoffman (eds),
'Review of Child Development Research', 1, New York:
Russell Sage Foundation.
ZOLA, I.K. (1975a), Culture and Symptoms: An Analysis of
Patients' Presenting Complaints, in C. Cox and A. Mead
(eds), 'A Sociology of Medical Practice', London:
Collier Macmillan.
ZOLA, I.K. (1975b), Medicine as an Institution of Social
Control, in C. Cox and A. Mead (eds), 'A Sociology of
Medical Practice', London: Collier Macmillan.

Index

Routledge Social Science Series

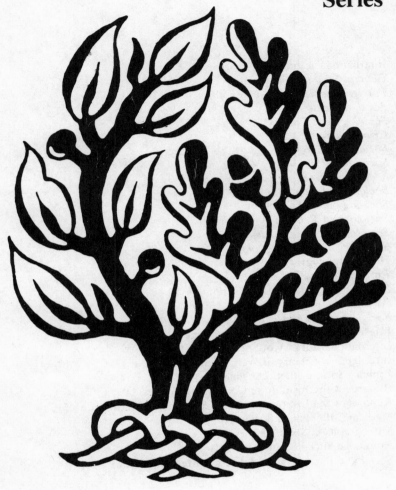

Routledge & Kegan Paul   London, Henley and Boston

39 Store Street, London WC1E 7DD
Broadway House, Newtown Road,
Henley-on-Thames, Oxon RG9 1EN
9 Park Street, Boston, Mass. 02108

Contents

*Authors wishing to submit manuscripts for any series in
this catalogue should send them to the Social Science Editor,
Routledge & Kegan Paul Ltd, 39 Store Street,
London WC1E 7DD*

●*Books so marked are available in paperback*
All books are in Metric Demy 8vo format (216 × 138mm approx.)

International Library of Sociology

General Editor   John Rex

GENERAL SOCIOLOGY

Barnsley, J. H. The Social Reality of Ethics. *464 pp.*
Brown, Robert. Explanation in Social Science. *208 pp.*
● Rules and Laws in Sociology. *192 pp.*
Bruford, W. H. Chekhov and His Russia. *A Sociological Study. 244 pp.*
Burton, F. and **Carlen, P.** Official Discourse. *On Discourse Analysis, Government Publications, Ideology. About 140 pp.*
Cain, Maureen E. Society and the Policeman's Role. *326 pp.*
●**Fletcher, Colin.** Beneath the Surface. *An Account of Three Styles of Sociological Research. 221 pp.*
Gibson, Quentin. The Logic of Social Enquiry. *240 pp.*
Glucksmann, M. Structuralist Analysis in Contemporary Social Thought. *212 pp.*
Gurvitch, Georges. Sociology of Law. *Foreword by Roscoe Pound. 264 pp.*
Hinkle, R. Founding Theory of American Sociology 1883-1915. *About 350 pp.*
Homans, George C. Sentiments and Activities. *336 pp.*
Johnson, Harry M. Sociology: *a Systematic Introduction. Foreword by Robert K. Merton. 710 pp.*
●**Keat, Russell** and **Urry, John.** Social Theory as Science. *278 pp.*
Mannheim, Karl. Essays on Sociology and Social Psychology. *Edited by Paul Keckskemeti. With Editorial Note by Adolph Lowe. 344 pp.*
Martindale, Don. The Nature and Types of Sociological Theory. *292 pp.*
●**Maus, Heinz.** A Short History of Sociology. *234 pp.*
Myrdal, Gunnar. Value in Social Theory: *A Collection of Essays on Methodology. Edited by Paul Streeten. 332 pp.*
Ogburn, William F. and **Nimkoff, Meyer F.** A Handbook of Sociology. *Preface by Karl Mannheim. 656 pp. 46 figures. 35 tables.*
Parsons, Talcott, and **Smelser, Neil J.** Economy and Society: *A Study in the Integration of Economic and Social Theory. 362 pp.*
Podgórecki, Adam. Practical Social Sciences. *About 200 pp.*
Raffel, S. Matters of Fact. *A Sociological Inquiry. 152 pp.*
●**Rex, John.** (Ed.) Approaches to Sociology. *Contributions by Peter Abell,* Sociology and the Demystification of the Modern World. *282 pp.*
●**Rex, John** (Ed.) Approaches to Sociology. *Contributions by Peter Abell, Frank Bechhofer, Basil Bernstein, Ronald Fletcher, David Frisby, Miriam Glucksmann, Peter Lassman, Herminio Martins, John Rex, Roland Robertson, John Westergaard and Jock Young. 302 pp.*
Rigby, A. Alternative Realities. *352 pp.*
Roche, M. Phenomenology, Language and the Social Sciences. *374 pp.*
Sahay, A. Sociological Analysis. *220 pp.*

Strasser, Hermann. The Normative Structure of Sociology. *Conservative and Emancipatory Themes in Social Thought. About 340 pp.*
Strong, P. Ceremonial Order of the Clinic. *About 250 pp.*
Urry, John. Reference Groups and the Theory of Revolution. *244 pp.*
Weinberg, E. Development of Sociology in the Soviet Union. *173 pp.*

FOREIGN CLASSICS OF SOCIOLOGY

● **Gerth, H. H.** and **Mills, C. Wright.** From Max Weber: *Essays in Sociology. 502 pp.*
● **Tönnies, Ferdinand.** Community and Association. *(Gemeinschaft and Gesellschaft.) Translated and Supplemented by Charles P. Loomis. Foreword by Pitirim A. Sorokin. 334 pp.*

SOCIAL STRUCTURE

Andreski, Stanislav. Military Organization and Society. *Foreword by Professor A. R. Radcliffe-Brown. 226 pp. 1 folder.*
Carlton, Eric. Ideology and Social Order. *Foreword by Professor Philip Abrahams. About 320 pp.*
Coontz, Sydney H. Population Theories and the Economic Interpretation. *202 pp.*
Coser, Lewis. The Functions of Social Conflict. *204 pp.*
Dickie-Clark, H. F. Marginal Situation: *A Sociological Study of a Coloured Group. 240 pp. 11 tables.*
Giner, S. and **Archer, M. S.** (Eds.). Contemporary Europe. *Social Structures and Cultural Patterns. 336 pp.*
● **Glaser, Barney** and **Strauss, Anselm L.** Status Passage. *A Formal Theory. 212 pp.*
Glass, D. V. (Ed.) Social Mobility in Britain. *Contributions by J. Berent, T. Bottomore, R. C. Chambers, J. Floud, D. V. Glass, J. R. Hall, H. T. Himmelweit, R. K. Kelsall, F. M. Martin, C. A. Moser, R. Mukherjee, and W. Ziegel. 420 pp.*
Kelsall, R. K. Higher Civil Servants in Britain: *From 1870 to the Present Day. 268 pp. 31 tables.*
● **Lawton, Denis.** Social Class, Language and Education. *192 pp.*
McLeish, John. The Theory of Social Change: *Four Views Considered. 128 pp.*
● **Marsh, David C.** The Changing Social Structure of England and Wales, 1871-1961. *Revised edition. 288 pp.*
Menzies, Ken. Talcott Parsons and the Social Image of Man. *About 208 pp.*
● **Mouzelis, Nicos.** Organization and Bureaucracy. *An Analysis of Modern Theories. 240 pp.*
Ossowski, Stanislaw. Class Structure in the Social Consciousness. *210 pp.*
● **Podgórecki, Adam.** Law and Society. *302 pp.*
Renner, Karl. Institutions of Private Law and Their Social Functions. *Edited, with an Introduction and Notes, by O. Kahn-Freud. Translated by Agnes Schwarzschild. 316 pp.*

Rex, J. and **Tomlinson, S.** Colonial Immigrants in a British City. *A Class Analysis. 368 pp.*

Smooha, S. Israel: Pluralism and Conflict. *472 pp.*

Wesolowski, W. Class, Strata and Power. *Trans. and with Introduction by G. Kolankiewicz. 160 pp.*

Zureik, E. Palestinians in Israel. *A Study in Internal Colonialism. 264 pp.*

SOCIOLOGY AND POLITICS

Acton, T. A. Gypsy Politics and Social Change. *316 pp.*

Burton, F. Politics of Legitimacy. *Struggles in a Belfast Community. 250 pp.*

Etzioni-Halevy, E. Political Manipulation and Administrative Power. *A Comparative Study. About 200 pp.*

● **Hechter, Michael.** Internal Colonialism. *The Celtic Fringe in British National Development, 1536–1966. 380 pp.*

Kornhauser, William. The Politics of Mass Society. *272 pp. 20 tables.*

Korpi, W. The Working Class in Welfare Capitalism. *Work, Unions and Politics in Sweden. 472 pp.*

Kroes, R. Soldiers and Students. *A Study of Right- and Left-wing Students. 174 pp.*

Martin, Roderick. Sociology of Power. *About 272 pp.*

Myrdal, Gunnar. The Political Element in the Development of Economic Theory. *Translated from the German by Paul Streeten. 282 pp.*

Wong, S.-L. Sociology and Socialism in Contemporary China. *160 pp.*

Wootton, Graham. Workers, Unions and the State. *188 pp.*

CRIMINOLOGY

Ancel, Marc. Social Defence: *A Modern Approach to Criminal Problems. Foreword by Leon Radzinowicz. 240 pp.*

Athens, L. Violent Criminal Acts and Actors. *About 150 pp.*

Cain, Maureen E. Society and the Policeman's Role. *326 pp.*

Cloward, Richard A. and **Ohlin, Lloyd E.** Delinquency and Opportunity: *A Theory of Delinquent Gangs. 248 pp.*

Downes, David M. The Delinquent Solution. *A Study in Subcultural Theory. 296 pp.*

Friedlander, Kate. The Psycho-Analytical Approach to Juvenile Delinquency: *Theory, Case Studies, Treatment. 320 pp.*

Gleuck, Sheldon and **Eleanor.** Family Environment and Delinquency. *With the statistical assistance of Rose W. Kneznek. 340 pp.*

Lopez-Rey, Manuel. Crime. *An Analytical Appraisal. 288 pp.*

Mannheim, Hermann. Comparative Criminology: *a Text Book. Two volumes. 442 pp. and 380 pp.*

Morris, Terence. The Criminal Area: *A Study in Social Ecology. Foreword by Hermann Mannheim. 232 pp. 25 tables. 4 maps.*

Podgorecki, A. and **Łos, M.** *Multidimensional Sociology. About 380 pp.*

Rock, Paul. Making People Pay. *338 pp.*

● **Taylor, Ian, Walton, Paul,** and **Young, Jock.** The New Criminology. *For a Social Theory of Deviance. 325 pp.*

● **Taylor, Ian, Walton, Paul** and **Young, Jock.** (Eds) Critical Criminology. *268 pp.*

SOCIAL PSYCHOLOGY

Bagley, Christopher. The Social Psychology of the Epileptic Child. *320 pp.*

Brittan, Arthur. Meanings and Situations. *224 pp.*

Carroll, J. Break-Out from the Crystal Palace. *200 pp.*

● **Fleming, C. M.** Adolescence: Its Social Psychology. *With an Introduction to recent findings from the fields of Anthropology, Physiology, Medicine, Psychometrics and Sociometry. 288 pp.*

●   The Social Psychology of Education: *An Introduction and Guide to Its Study. 136 pp.*

Linton, Ralph. The Cultural Background of Personality. *132 pp.*

● **Mayo, Elton.** The Social Problems of an Industrial Civilization. *With an Appendix on the Political Problem. 180 pp.*

Ottaway, A. K. C. Learning Through Group Experience. *176 pp.*

Plummer, Ken. Sexual Stigma. *An Interactionist Account. 254 pp.*

● **Rose, Arnold M.** (Ed.) Human Behaviour and Social Processes: *an Interactionist Approach. Contributions by Arnold M. Rose, Ralph H. Turner, Anselm Strauss, Everett C. Hughes, E. Franklin Frazier, Howard S. Becker et al. 696 pp.*

Smelser, Neil J. Theory of Collective Behaviour. *448 pp.*

Stephenson, Geoffrey M. The Development of Conscience. *128 pp.*

Young, Kimball. Handbook of Social Psychology. *658 pp. 16 figures. 10 tables.*

SOCIOLOGY OF THE FAMILY

Bell, Colin R. Middle Class Families: *Social and Geographical Mobility. 224 pp.*

Burton, Lindy. Vulnerable Children. *272 pp.*

Gavron, Hannah. The Captive Wife: *Conflicts of Household Mothers. 190 pp.*

George, Victor and **Wilding, Paul.** Motherless Families. *248 pp.*

Klein, Josephine. Samples from English Cultures.
1. Three Preliminary Studies and Aspects of Adult Life in England. *447 pp.*
2. Child-Rearing Practices and Index. *247 pp.*

Klein, Viola. The Feminine Character. *History of an Ideology. 244 pp.*

McWhinnie, Alexina M. Adopted Children. *How They Grow Up. 304 pp.*

● **Morgan, D. H. J.** Social Theory and the Family. *About 320 pp.*

● **Myrdal, Alva** and **Klein, Viola.** Women's Two Roles: *Home and Work. 238 pp. 27 tables.*

Parsons, Talcott and **Bales, Robert F.** Family: Socialization and Inter-action Process. *In collaboration with James Olds, Morris Zelditch and Philip E. Slater. 456 pp. 50 figures and tables.*

SOCIAL SERVICES

Bastide, Roger. The Sociology of Mental Disorder. *Translated from the French by Jean McNeil. 260 pp.*

Carlebach, Julius. Caring For Children in Trouble. *266 pp.*

George, Victor. Foster Care. *Theory and Practice. 234 pp.*
  Social Security: *Beveridge and After. 258 pp.*

George, V. and **Wilding, P.** Motherless Families. *248 pp.*

● **Goetschius, George W.** Working with Community Groups. *256 pp.*

Goetschius, George W. and **Tash, Joan.** Working with Unattached Youth. *416 pp.*

Heywood, Jean S. Children in Care. *The Development of the Service for the Deprived Child. Third revised edition. 284 pp.*

King, Roy D., Ranes, Norma V. and **Tizard, Jack.** Patterns of Residen-tial Care. *356 pp.*

Leigh, John. Young People and Leisure. *256 pp.*

● **Mays, John.** (Ed.) Penelope Hall's Social Services of England and Wales. *About 324 pp.*

Morris, Mary. Voluntary Work and the Welfare State. *300 pp.*

Nokes, P. L. The Professional Task in Welfare Practice. *152 pp.*

Timms, Noel. Psychiatric Social Work in Great Britain (1939-1962). *280 pp.*

● Social Casework: *Principles and Practice. 256 pp.*

SOCIOLOGY OF EDUCATION

Banks, Olive. Parity and Prestige in English Secondary Education: a Study in Educational Sociology. *272 pp.*

● **Blyth, W. A. L.** English Primary Education. *A Sociological Description.* 2. Background. *168 pp.*

Collier, K. G. The Social Purposes of Education: *Personal and Social Values in Education. 268 pp.*

Evans, K. M. Sociometry and Education. *158 pp.*

● **Ford, Julienne.** Social Class and the Comprehensive School. *192 pp.*

Foster, P. J. Education and Social Change in Ghana. *336 pp. 3 maps.*

Fraser, W. R. Education and Society in Modern France. *150 pp.*

Grace, Gerald R. Role Conflict and the Teacher. *150 pp.*

Hans, Nicholas. New Trends in Education in the Eighteenth Century. *278 pp. 19 tables.*

● Comparative Education: *A Study of Educational Factors and Tra-ditions. 360 pp.*

● **Hargreaves, David.** Interpersonal Relations and Education. *432 pp.*

● Social Relations in a Secondary School. *240 pp.*

  School Organization and Pupil Involvement. *A Study of Secondary Schools.*

7

● **Mannheim, Karl** and **Stewart, W.A.C.** An Introduction to the Sociology of Education. *206 pp.*

● **Musgrove, F.** Youth and the Social Order. *176 pp.*

● **Ottaway, A. K. C.** Education and Society: An Introduction to the Sociology of Education. *With an Introduction by W. O. Lester Smith. 212 pp.*

Peers, Robert. Adult Education: *A Comparative Study. Revised edition. 398 pp.*

Stratta, Erica. The Education of Borstal Boys. *A Study of their Educational Experiences prior to, and during, Borstal Training. 256 pp.*

● **Taylor, P. H., Reid, W. A.** and **Holley, B. J.** The English Sixth Form. *A Case Study in Curriculum Research. 198 pp.*

SOCIOLOGY OF CULTURE

Eppel, E. M. and **M.** Adolescents and Morality: *A Study of some Moral Values and Dilemmas of Working Adolescents in the Context of a changing Climate of Opinion. Foreword by W. J. H. Sprott. 268 pp. 39 tables.*

● **Fromm, Erich.** The Fear of Freedom. *286 pp.*
●   The Sane Society. *400 pp.*

Johnson, L. The Cultural Critics. *From Matthew Arnold to Raymond Williams. 233 pp.*

Mannheim, Karl. Essays on the Sociology of Culture. *Edited by Ernst Mannheim in co-operation with Paul Kecskemeti. Editorial Note by Adolph Lowe. 280 pp.*

Zijderfeld, A. C. On Clichés. *The Supersedure of Meaning by Function in Modernity. About 132 pp.*

SOCIOLOGY OF RELIGION

Argyle, Michael and **Beit-Hallahmi, Benjamin.** The Social Psychology of Religion. *About 256 pp.*

Glasner, Peter E. The Sociology of Secularisation. *A Critique of a Concept. About 180 pp.*

Hall, J. R. The Ways Out. *Utopian Communal Groups in an Age of Babylon. 280 pp.*

Ranson, S., Hinings, B. and **Bryman, A.** Clergy, Ministers and Priests. *216 pp.*

Stark, Werner. The Sociology of Religion. *A Study of Christendom.*
Volume II. *Sectarian Religion. 368 pp.*
Volume III. *The Universal Church. 464 pp.*
Volume IV. *Types of Religious Man. 352 pp.*
Volume V. *Types of Religious Culture. 464 pp.*

Turner, B. S. Weber and Islam. *216 pp.*

Watt, W. Montgomery. Islam and the Integration of Society. *320 pp.*

SOCIOLOGY OF ART AND LITERATURE

Jarvie, Ian C. Towards a Sociology of the Cinema. *A Comparative Essay on the Structure and Functioning of a Major Entertainment Industry. 405 pp.*

Rust, Frances S. Dance in Society. *An Analysis of the Relationships between the Social Dance and Society in England from the Middle Ages to the Present Day. 256 pp. 8 pp. of plates.*

Schücking, L. L. The Sociology of Literary Taste. *112 pp.*

Wolff, Janet. Hermeneutic Philosophy and the Sociology of Art. *150 pp.*

SOCIOLOGY OF KNOWLEDGE

Diesing, P. Patterns of Discovery in the Social Sciences. *262 pp.*

● **Douglas, J. D.** (Ed.) Understanding Everyday Life. *370 pp.*

Glasner, B. Essential Interactionism. *About 220 pp.*

● **Hamilton, P.** Knowledge and Social Structure. *174 pp.*

Jarvie, I. C. Concepts and Society. *232 pp.*

Mannheim, Karl. Essays on the Sociology of Knowledge. *Edited by Paul Kecskemeti. Editorial Note by Adolph Lowe. 353 pp.*

Remmling, Gunter W. The Sociology of Karl Mannheim. *With a Bibliographical Guide to the Sociology of Knowledge, Ideological Analysis, and Social Planning. 255 pp.*

Remmling, Gunter W. (Ed.) Towards the Sociology of Knowledge. *Origin and Development of a Sociological Thought Style. 463 pp.*

URBAN SOCIOLOGY

Aldridge, M. The British New Towns. *A Programme Without a Policy. About 250 pp.*

Ashworth, William. The Genesis of Modern British Town Planning: *A Study in Economic and Social History of the Nineteenth and Twentieth Centuries. 288 pp.*

Brittan, A. The Privatised World. *196 pp.*

Cullingworth, J. B. Housing Needs and Planning Policy: *A Restatement of the Problems of Housing Need and 'Overspill' in England and Wales. 232 pp. 44 tables. 8 maps.*

Dickinson, Robert E. City and Region: *A Geographical Interpretation. 608 pp. 125 figures.*

The West European City: *A Geographical Interpretation. 600 pp. 129 maps. 29 plates.*

Humphreys, Alexander J. New Dubliners: *Urbanization and the Irish Family. Foreword by George C. Homans. 304 pp.*

Jackson, Brian. Working Class Community: *Some General Notions raised by a Series of Studies in Northern England. 192 pp.*

● **Mann, P. H.** An Approach to Urban Sociology. *240 pp.*

Mellor, J. R. Urban Sociology in an Urbanized Society. *326 pp.*

Morris, R. N. and **Mogey, J.** The Sociology of Housing. *Studies at Berinsfield. 232 pp. 4 pp. plates.*

Rosser, C. and **Harris, C.** The Family and Social Change. *A Study of Family and Kinship in a South Wales Town. 352 pp. 8 maps.*

● **Stacey, Margaret, Batsone, Eric, Bell, Colin** and **Thurcott, Anne.** Power, Persistence and Change. *A Second Study of Banbury. 196 pp.*

RURAL SOCIOLOGY

Mayer, Adrian C. Peasants in the Pacific. *A Study of Fiji Indian Rural Society. 248 pp. 20 plates.*

Williams, W. M. The Sociology of an English Village: *Gosforth. 272 pp. 12 figures. 13 tables.*

SOCIOLOGY OF INDUSTRY AND DISTRIBUTION

Dunkerley, David. The Foreman. *Aspects of Task and Structure. 192 pp.*

Eldridge, J. E. T. Industrial Disputes. *Essays in the Sociology of Industrial Relations. 288 pp.*

Hollowell, Peter G. The Lorry Driver. *272 pp.*

● **Oxaal, I., Barnett, T.** and **Booth, D.** (Eds) Beyond the Sociology of Development. *Economy and Society in Latin America and Africa. 295 pp.*

Smelser, Neil J. Social Change in the Industrial Revolution: *An Application of Theory to the Lancashire Cotton Industry, 1770–1840. 468 pp. 12 figures. 14 tables.*

Watson, T. J. The Personnel Managers. *A Study in the Sociology of Work and Employment. 262 pp.*

ANTHROPOLOGY

Brandel-Syrier, Mia. Reeftown Elite. *A Study of Social Mobility in a Modern African Community on the Reef. 376 pp.*

Dickie-Clark, H. F. The Marginal Situation. *A Sociological Study of a Coloured Group. 236 pp.*

Dube, S. C. Indian Village. *Foreword by Morris Edward Opler. 276 pp. 4 plates.*

India's Changing Villages: *Human Factors in Community Development. 260 pp. 8 plates. 1 map.*

Firth, Raymond. Malay Fishermen. *Their Peasant Economy. 420 pp. 17 pp. plates.*

Gulliver, P. H. Social Control in an African Society: a Study of the Arusha, Agricultural Masai of Northern Tanganyika. *320 pp. 8 plates. 10 figures.*

Family Herds. *288 pp.*

Jarvie, Ian C. The Revolution in Anthropology. *268 pp.*

Little, Kenneth L. Mende of Sierra Leone. *308 pp. and folder.*

Negroes in Britain. *With a New Introduction and Contemporary Study by Leonard Bloom. 320 pp.*

Madan, G. R. Western Sociologists on Indian Society. *Marx, Spencer, Weber, Durkheim, Pareto. 384 pp.*

Mayer, A. C. Peasants in the Pacific. *A Study of Fiji Indian Rural Society. 248 pp.*

Meer, Fatima. Race and Suicide in South Africa. *325 pp.*

Smith, Raymond T. The Negro Family in British Guiana: *Family Structure and Social Status in the Villages. With a Foreword by Meyer Fortes. 314 pp. 8 plates. 1 figure. 4 maps.*

SOCIOLOGY AND PHILOSOPHY

Barnsley, John H. The Social Reality of Ethics. *A Comparative Analysis of Moral Codes. 448 pp.*

Diesing, Paul. Patterns of Discovery in the Social Sciences. *362 pp.*

● **Douglas, Jack D.** (Ed.) Understanding Everyday Life. *Toward the Reconstruction of Sociological Knowledge. Contributions by Alan F. Blum, Aaron W. Cicourel, Norman K. Denzin, Jack D. Douglas, John Heeren, Peter McHugh, Peter K. Manning, Melvin Power, Matthew Speier, Roy Turner, D. Lawrence Wieder, Thomas P. Wilson and Don H. Zimmerman. 370 pp.*

Gorman, Robert A. The Dual Vision. *Alfred Schutz and the Myth of Phenomenological Social Science. About 300 pp.*

Jarvie, Ian C. Concepts and Society. *216 pp.*

Kilminster, R. Praxis and Method. *A Sociological Dialogue with Lukács, Gramsci and the early Frankfurt School. About 304 pp.*

● **Pelz, Werner.** The Scope of Understanding in Sociology. *Towards a More Radical Reorientation in the Social Humanistic Sciences. 283 pp.*

Roche, Maurice. Phenomenology, Language and the Social Sciences. *371 pp.*

Sahay, Arun. Sociological Analysis. *212 pp.*

Slater, P. Origin and Significance of the Frankfurt School. *A Marxist Perspective. About 192 pp.*

Spurling, L. Phenomenology and the Social World. *The Philosophy of Merleau-Ponty and its Relation to the Social Sciences. 222 pp.*

Wilson, H. T. The American Ideology. *Science, Technology and Organization as Modes of Rationality. 368 pp.*

International Library of Anthropology

General Editor Adam Kuper

Ahmed, A. S. Millenium and Charisma Among Pathans. *A Critical Essay in Social Anthropology. 192 pp.*
  Pukhtun Economy and Society. *About 360 pp.*

Brown, Paula. The Chimbu. *A Study of Change in the New Guinea Highlands. 151 pp.*

Foner, N. Jamaica Farewell. *200 pp.*

Gudeman, Stephen. Relationships, Residence and the Individual. *A Rural Panamanian Community. 288 pp. 11 plates, 5 figures, 2 maps, 10 tables.*

   The Demise of a Rural Economy. *From Subsistence to Capitalism in a Latin American Village. 160 pp.*

Hamnett, Ian. Chieftainship and Legitimacy. *An Anthropological Study of Executive Law in Lesotho. 163 pp.*

Hanson, F. Allan. Meaning in Culture. *127 pp.*

Humphreys, S. C. Anthropology and the Greeks. *288 pp.*

Karp, I. Fields of Change Among the Iteso of Kenya. *140 pp.*

Lloyd, P. C. Power and Independence. *Urban Africans' Perception of Social Inequality. 264 pp.*

Parry, J. P. Caste and Kinship in Kangra. *352 pp. Illustrated.*

Pettigrew, Joyce. Robber Noblemen. *A Study of the Political System of the Sikh Jats. 284 pp.*

Street, Brian V. The Savage in Literature. *Representations of 'Primitive' Society in English Fiction, 1858–1920. 207 pp.*

Van Den Berghe, Pierre L. Power and Privilege at an African University. *278 pp.*

International Library of Social Policy

General Editor Kathleen Jones

Bayley, M. Mental Handicap and Community Care. *426 pp.*

Bottoms, A. E. and **McClean, J. D.** Defendants in the Criminal Process. *284 pp.*

Butler, J. R. Family Doctors and Public Policy. *208 pp.*

Davies, Martin. Prisoners of Society. *Attitudes and Aftercare. 204 pp.*

Gittus, Elizabeth. Flats, Families and the Under-Fives. *285 pp.*

Holman, Robert. Trading in Children. *A Study of Private Fostering. 355 pp.*

Jeffs, A. Young People and the Youth Service. *About 180 pp.*

Jones, Howard, and **Cornes, Paul.** Open Prisons. *288 pp.*

Jones, Kathleen. History of the Mental Health Service. *428 pp.*

Jones, Kathleen, with **Brown, John, Cunningham, W. J., Roberts, Julian** and **Williams, Peter.** Opening the Door. *A Study of New Policies for the Mentally Handicapped. 278 pp.*

Karn, Valerie. Retiring to the Seaside. *About 280 pp. 2 maps. Numerous tables.*

King, R. D. and **Elliot, K. W.** Albany: Birth of a Prison—End of an Era. *394 pp.*

Thomas, J. E. The English Prison Officer since 1850: *A Study in Conflict.* *258 pp.*

Walton, R. G. Women in Social Work. *303 pp.*

● **Woodward, J.** To Do the Sick No Harm. *A Study of the British Voluntary Hospital System to 1875. 234 pp.*

International Library of Welfare and Philosophy

General Editors Noel Timms and David Watson

● **McDermott, F. E.** (Ed.) Self-Determination in Social Work. *A Collection of Essays on Self-determination and Related Concepts by Philosophers and Social Work Theorists. Contributors: F. B. Biestek, S. Bernstein, A. Keith-Lucas, D. Sayer, H. H. Perelman, C. Whittington, R. F. Stalley, F. E. McDermott, I. Berlin, H. J. McCloskey, H. L. A. Hart, J. Wilson, A. I. Melden, S. I. Benn. 254 pp.*

● **Plant, Raymond.** Community and Ideology. *104 pp.*

Ragg, Nicholas M. People Not Cases. *A Philosophical Approach to Social Work. About 250 pp.*

● **Timms, Noel** and **Watson, David.** (Eds) Talking About Welfare. *Readings in Philosophy and Social Policy. Contributors: T. H. Marshall, R. B. Brandt, G. H. von Wright, K. Nielsen, M. Cranston, R. M. Titmuss, R. S. Downie, E. Telfer, D. Donnison, J. Benson, P. Leonard, A. Keith-Lucas, D. Walsh, I. T. Ramsey. 320 pp.*

● (Eds). Philosophy in Social Work. *250 pp.*

● **Weale, A.** Equality and Social Policy. *164 pp.*

Primary Socialization, Language and Education

General Editor Basil Bernstein

Adlam, Diana S., *with the assistance of Geoffrey Turner and Lesley Lineker.* Code in Context. *About 272 pp.*

Bernstein, Basil. Class, Codes and Control. *3 volumes.*

● 1. *Theoretical Studies Towards a Sociology of Language. 254 pp.*

2. *Applied Studies Towards a Sociology of Language. 377 pp.*

● 3. *Towards a Theory of Educational Transmission. 167 pp.*

Brandis, W. and **Bernstein, B.** Selection and Control. *176 pp.*

Brandis, Walter and **Henderson, Dorothy.** Social Class, Language and Communication. *288 pp.*

Cook-Gumperz, Jenny. Social Control and Socialization. *A Study of Class Differences in the Language of Maternal Control. 290 pp.*

● **Gahagan, D. M** and **G. A.** Talk Reform. *Exploration in Language for Infant School Children. 160 pp.*

Hawkins, P. R. Social Class, the Nominal Group and Verbal Strategies. *About 220 pp.*

Robinson, W. P. and **Rackstraw, Susan D. A.** A Question of Answers. *2 volumes. 192 pp. and 180 pp.*

Turner, Geoffrey J. and **Mohan, Bernard A.** A Linguistic Description and Computer Programme for Children's Speech. *208 pp.*

Reports of the Institute of Community Studies

Baker, J. The Neighbourhood Advice Centre. A Community Project in Camden. *320 pp.*

● **Cartwright, Ann.** Patients and their Doctors. *A Study of General Practice. 304 pp.*

Dench, Geoff. Maltese in London. *A Case-study in the Erosion of Ethnic Consciousness. 302 pp.*

Jackson, Brian and **Marsden, Dennis.** Education and the Working Class: *Some General Themes raised by a Study of 88 Working-class Children in a Northern Industrial City. 268 pp. 2 folders.*

Marris, Peter. The Experience of Higher Education. *232 pp. 27 tables.*
● Loss and Change. *192 pp.*

Marris, Peter and **Rein, Martin.** Dilemmas of Social Reform. *Poverty and Community Action in the United States. 256 pp.*

Marris, Peter and **Somerset, Anthony.** African Businessmen. *A Study of Entrepreneurship and Development in Keyna. 256 pp.*

Mills, Richard. Young Outsiders: *a Study in Alternative Communities. 216 pp.*

Runciman, W. G. Relative Deprivation and Social Justice. *A Study of Attitudes to Social Inequality in Twentieth-Century England. 352 pp.*

Willmott, Peter. Adolescent Boys in East London. *230 pp.*

Willmott, Peter and **Young, Michael.** Family and Class in a London Suburb. *202 pp. 47 tables.*

Young, Michael and **McGeeney, Patrick.** Learning Begins at Home. *A Study of a Junior School and its Parents. 128 pp.*

Young, Michael and **Willmott, Peter.** Family and Kinship in East London. *Foreword by Richard M. Titmuss. 252 pp. 39 tables.*
The Symmetrical Family. *410 pp.*

Reports of the Institute for Social Studies in Medical Care

Cartwright, Ann, Hockey, Lisbeth and **Anderson, John J.** Life Before Death. *310 pp.*

Dunnell, Karen and **Cartwright, Ann.** Medicine Takers, Prescribers and Hoarders. *190 pp.*

Farrell, C. My Mother Said. . . . *A Study of the Way Young People Learned About Sex and Birth Control. 200 pp.*

Medicine, Illness and Society

General Editor W. M. Williams

Hall, David J. Social Relations & Innovation. *Changing the State of Play in Hospitals. 232 pp.*

Hall, David J., and **Stacey, M.** (Eds) Beyond Separation. *234 pp.*

Robinson, David. The Process of Becoming Ill. *142 pp.*

Stacey, Margaret *et al.* Hospitals, Children and Their Families. *The Report of a Pilot Study. 202 pp.*

Stimson G. V. and **Webb, B.** Going to See the Doctor. *The Consultation Process in General Practice. 155 pp.*

Monographs in Social Theory

General Editor Arthur Brittan

● **Barnes, B.** Scientific Knowledge and Sociological Theory. *192 pp.*

Bauman, Zygmunt. Culture as Praxis. *204 pp.*

● **Dixon, Keith.** Sociological Theory. *Pretence and Possibility. 142 pp.*

Meltzer, B. N., Petras, J. W. and **Reynolds, L. T.** Symbolic Interactionism. *Genesis, Varieties and Criticisms. 144 pp.*

● **Smith, Anthony D.** The Concept of Social Change. *A Critique of the Functionalist Theory of Social Change. 208 pp.*

Routledge Social Science Journals

The British Journal of Sociology. *Editor – Angus Stewart; Associate Editor – Leslie Sklair. Vol. 1, No. 1 – March 1950 and Quarterly. Roy. 8vo. All back issues available. An international journal publishing original papers in the field of sociology and related areas.*

Community Work. *Edited by David Jones and Marjorie Mayo. 1973. Published annually.*

Economy and Society. *Vol. 1, No. 1. February 1972 and Quarterly. Metric Roy. 8vo. A journal for all social scientists covering sociology, philosophy, anthropology, economics and history. All back numbers available.*

Ethnic and Racial Studies. *Editor – John Stone. Vol. 1 – 1978. Published quarterly.*

Religion. Journal of Religion and Religions. *Chairman of Editorial Board, Ninian Smart. Vol. 1, No. 1, Spring 1971. A journal with an inter-disciplinary approach to the study of the phenomena of religion. All back numbers available.*

Sociology of Health and Illness. *A Journal of Medical Sociology. Editor – Alan Davies; Associate Editor – Ray Jobling. Vol. 1, Spring 1979. Published 3 times per annum.*

Year Book of Social Policy in Britain, The. *Edited by Kathleen Jones. 1971. Published annually.*

Social and Psychological Aspects of Medical Practice

Editor   Trevor Silverstone

Lader, Malcolm. Psychophysiology of Mental Illness. *280 pp.*
● **Silverstone, Trevor** and **Turner, Paul.** Drug Treatment in Psychiatry. *Revised edition. 256 pp.*
Whiteley, J. S. and **Gordon, J.** Group Approaches in Psychiatry. *256 pp.*

Printed in Great Britain by
Lowe & Brydone Printers Limited, Thetford, Norfolk